ATLAS OF EXTRAOCULAR MUSCLE SURGERY

Second Edition

John A. Dyer, M.D., M.S.
(Ophthalmology)

*Professor of Ophthalmology, Mayo Medical School;
Consultant, Department of Ophthalmology, Mayo Clinic
and Mayo Foundation; Rochester, Minnesota*

David A. Lee, M.D., M.S.
(Ophthalmology)

*Instructor in Ophthalmology, Mayo Medical School;
Fellow in Ophthalmology, Mayo Graduate School of Medicine;
Rochester, Minnesota*

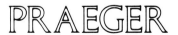

PRAEGER SPECIAL STUDIES • PRAEGER SCIENTIFIC

New York • Philadelphia • Eastbourne, UK
Toronto • Hong Kong • Tokyo • Sydney

Dedicated

to my devoted wife

Rena

whose patient encouragement made
easier the accomplishment of this work

J.A.D.

Library of Congress Cataloging in Publication Data

Dyer, John A. (John Allen)
Atlas of extraocular muscle surgery.

Bibliography: p.
Includes index.
1. Strabismus—Surgery—Atlases. 2. Eye—Muscles—
Surgery—Atlases. I. Lee, David A. II. Title. [DNLM:
1. Oculomotor Muscles—surgery—atlases. WW 17 D996a]
RE771.D94 1984 617.7′62 84-18090
ISBN 0-03-000837-9 (alk. paper)

While care has been taken to maintain the accuracy of the information contained in this volume, the authors, editors, and publisher cannot accept any legal responsibility for errors or omissions, or for consequences arising from the use of the information contained herein and make no warranty, express or implied, with respect to the materials presented in this volume.

Published in 1984 by Praeger Publishers
CBS Educational and Professional Publishing
a Division of CBS Inc.
521 Fifth Avenue, New York, NY 10175 USA
© 1984 by Mayo Foundation

456789 052 98765432
Printed in the United States of America
on acid-free paper

Preface

At the insistence of my residents and because of the lack of a practical guide to ocular muscle surgery, this text was undertaken. The ideas expressed and the operations illustrated and described are those which I have formulated during several years of practicing the subspecialty of strabismus (squint) surgery. Undoubtedly my opinions have been influenced by many lectures, articles, and personal communications, and I extend my appreciation to those authors whose ideas or techniques have contributed to my own. However, since no single procedure or thought described or expressed herein could be identified necessarily with a particular surgeon, the bibliography has been chosen to provide for supplementary study and not to indicate sources.

In attempting to give some concrete suggestions as to how much surgery to do for a given defect, I have been guided by my own experience with procedures that have been effective for me. The description of those procedures constitutes the primary aim of this text.

Essential to the success of any surgical atlas is the accuracy of the illustrations, and I owe a debt of gratitude to Mr. Denis Lee, formerly of the Section of Medical Illustrations, and to Mr. John Hutcheson, Section of Medical Graphics, who provided additional surgical illustrations. My appreciation goes to Mrs. LeAnn Stee, Section of Publications, for her organization of the material in this text. Especially I wish to thank David A. Lee, M.D., for assisting me in the revision of this atlas, Allan B. Gould, Jr., M.D., for the chapter on anesthesia, and John Samples, M.D., University of Oregon at Portland (formerly from the Mayo Clinic), for assisting in the preparation of the flowcharts.

John A. Dyer

Contents

Contents

Part Three   *Additional Considerations for Each Operation*

Part Four   *Indications for and Types of Operative Procedures*

Part Five   *Complications and Technical Errors*

Part Six   *Anesthesia for Strabismus Surgery*
by Allan B. Gould, Jr., M.D.

PART ONE

Surgical Anatomy

Tenon's Capsule

This relatively dense, translucent, minimally vascular, fibroelastic connective tissue capsule envelops the posterior four fifths of the globe and the extraocular muscles in the anterior orbit, separating them from the orbital fat. Its smooth and glistening nature makes it an ideal surface to allow maximal freedom of movement of one fascial plane against another during rotation of the globe. A potential space exists between these fascial planes. Tenon's capsule is divided into anterior and posterior portions. The anterior portion of Tenon's capsule extends from the four rectus muscle penetrations posteriorly and fuses with the conjunctiva at the limbus anteriorly. The posterior portion of Tenon's capsule lies between the rectus muscle penetrations and the optic nerve and is composed of the fibrous muscle sheaths and intermuscular membranes. A free space exists between posterior Tenon's capsule and the sclera except for the points of exit of the vortex veins near the equator, the insertions of the oblique muscles, and the points of entrance of the posterior ciliary arteries and nerves. The attachments of the muscle fibers to the sheaths are quite firm; thus, the muscles will not retract excessively when severed (lost muscle), unless a large resection with clearing of the capsular tissue about the muscle has been performed. Most extraocular muscle surgery is done under the anterior portion of Tenon's capsule and in the plane of the posterior portion of Tenon's capsule.

The capsules of very young patients are quite pronounced and can be delineated rather easily from conjunctiva, whereas those of adults are thinner and more adherent to the conjunctiva. Care must be taken, in the case of young patients, to close the conjunctiva as well as Tenon's capsule; otherwise, a postoperative capsular cyst may occur.

Vortex Veins

The lateral (temporal) vortex veins are of clinical importance in ocular muscle surgery. The superior temporal vortex vein (Fig. 1) exits obliquely from the sclera about 8 mm behind the equator, close to the insertion of the superior oblique muscle. The vein is easier to identify if the surgeon approaches the superior oblique tendon along the nasal side of the superior rectus muscle. The inferior temporal vortex vein (Fig. 1) is more anterior and leaves the sclera obliquely about 5.5 mm posterior to the equator and about 7 to 8 mm below the plane of insertion of the inferior oblique muscle. Because of their exit positions and oblique courses through the sclera, the veins may be severed or ligated in the process of sewing a superior oblique tuck in position or during a recession of the inferior oblique muscle.

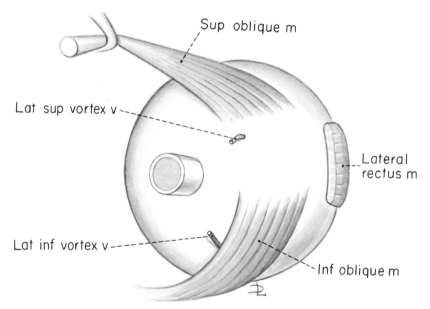

Figure 1. Lateral superior and inferior vortex veins (right eye).

Motor Innervation to the Extraocular Muscles

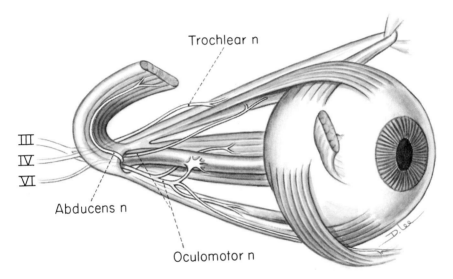

Figure 2. Motor nerve supply to extraocular muscles (right eye).

The motor nerve supply to the extraocular muscles is illustrated in Figure 2 and described in Table 1.

Table 1. Motor Nerves Supplying Extraocular Muscles

Muscle	Motor Nerve	Entrance of Nerve into Muscle
Medial rectus	Inferior division of N III	Lateral surface of muscle, near junction of middle and posterior thirds
Inferior rectus	Inferior division of N III	Upper side of muscle, near junction of middle and posterior thirds
Lateral rectus	N VI	Medial aspect of muscle, near center
Superior rectus	Superior division of N III	At junction of middle and posterior thirds of muscle
Inferior oblique	Inferior division of N III	Superior surface of muscle, near center
Superior oblique	N IV	Upper surface of muscle, near outer border (anterior branch enters at junction of middle and posterior thirds of muscle; posterior branch enters muscle about 8 mm from its own origin)

Blood Supply to the Extraocular Muscles

The arteries supplying the extraocular muscles are illustrated in Figure 3 and listed in Table 2.

The anterior ciliary arteries, arising from the muscular branches of the ophthalmic artery and piercing the sclera in front of the rectus muscle insertions (Fig. 4 and Table 2), enter the iris to form its major arterial circle. At least a portion of this blood supply must be preserved during muscle surgery to prevent segmental atrophy of the iris. Only half of the superior and inferior rectus muscles should be freed from the scleral insertions for muscle-transposition operations unless a horizontal rectus muscle is left intact.

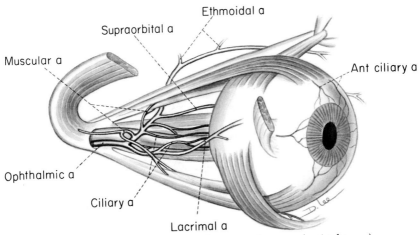

Figure 3. Arterial supply of extraocular muscles (right eye).

Table 2. Arteries Supplying Extraocular Muscles

Muscle	Artery	Divisions of Artery at Point of Scleral Insertion of Muscle
Medial rectus	Inferior muscular branch of ophthalmic	Usually two
Inferior rectus	Inferior muscular branch of ophthalmic	Usually two
Lateral rectus	Lacrimal	Usually one
Superior rectus	Superior muscular branch of ophthalmic	Two
Inferior oblique	Infraorbital and inferior muscular branches of ophthalmic	None
Superior oblique	Superior muscular branch of ophthalmic	None

Table 3. Scleral Insertions of Rectus Muscles: Pertinent Measurements

| | Measurements (mm) | | | |
| | Scleral Insertion to Anterior Limbus | Tendinous Portion of Muscle | | |
Muscle		Length	Width	Comment
Medial rectus	5.3	4.0	11.3	Slightly concave insertion
Inferior rectus	6.8	6.0	10.5	Nasal edge of insertion nearly 5.5 mm from medial rectus insertion
Lateral rectus	6.9	9.0	10.1	Slightly concave insertion; lower edge about 7.0 mm from inferior rectus insertion
Superior rectus	7.9	6.0	11.5	Nearly 6.5 mm from lateral rectus insertion and about 7.0 mm from that of medial rectus

Data from Apt, L.: An anatomical reevaluation of rectus muscle insertions. Trans. Am. Ophthalmol. Soc. 78:365–375, 1980.

Rectus Muscle Insertions and Measurements

Pertinent measurements relative to the scleral insertions of the rectus muscles are illustrated in Figure 4 and listed in Table 3.

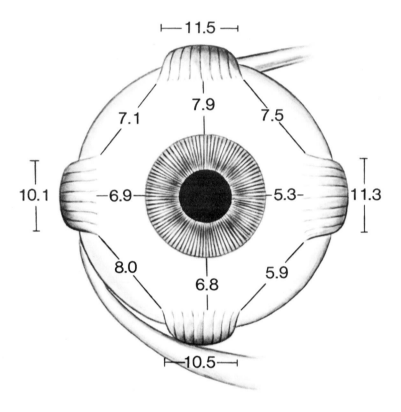

Figure 4. Muscle insertions and measurements (right eye).

Relationships and Actions of the Extraocular Muscles

Medial Rectus Muscle

The largest of the extraocular muscles, the medial rectus muscle arises on the inner side of and below the optic foramen, passes along the medial orbital wall, and inserts into the sclera 5.3 mm from the limbus.

Its action is purely adduction, and on convergence both medial rectus muscles act simultaneously.

Inferior Rectus Muscle

Arising below the optic foramen from the middle slip of the lower common ring tendon, this is the shortest of the rectus muscles. Passing forward along the orbital floor, it makes an angle of 23 degrees with the visual axis and inserts into the sclera 6.8 mm from the limbus. The inferior oblique muscle crosses beneath it, the sheaths of the two muscles being united to form Lockwood's ligament. Below the inferior rectus muscle lies the orbital floor, but anteriorly the muscle is separated from the orbital plate of the superior part of the maxilla by orbital fat. The nerve to the inferior oblique muscle courses in front of the lateral border of the inferior rectus muscle or between it and the lateral rectus muscle.

The primary action is depression when the eye is abducted. Secondarily, it aids in adduction and extorts the eye when it is turned inward.

Lateral Rectus Muscle

The lateral rectus muscle arises from both the lower and upper parts of the common ring tendon, from those portions that bridge the superior orbital fissure. It passes forward along the lateral orbital wall, turns inward toward the globe through Tenon's capsule, and inserts 6.9 mm from the limbus. Along the anterior part of the muscle, but above it, are the lacrimal artery and nerve. The lacrimal gland lies anteriorly. Beneath the muscle is the orbital floor, and anteriorly the tendinous condensation of the inferior oblique muscle passes beneath it to insert into the sclera about 10 mm from the lateral rectus insertion. Between the lateral rectus and inferior rectus muscles is the nerve to the inferior oblique muscle. Laterally the lateral rectus muscle lies against the periorbita posteriorly; more anteriorly some perimuscular fat intervenes.

Its action is purely abduction.

Superior Rectus Muscle

Arising from the upper part of the annulus of Zinn, laterally and above the optic foramen, and from the sheath of the optic nerve, the superior rectus muscle courses forward and outward, underlying the levator, at an angle of 23 degrees with the visual axis, penetrates Tenon's capsule, and inserts into the sclera 7.9 mm from the limbus; the insertion is oblique so that it is nearer the cornea nasally than temporally. Above, the muscle is in close approximation to the levator and frontal nerves, which separate it from the orbital roof. Below the muscle, anteriorly, are the reflected tendon of the superior oblique muscle and the globe.

The primary action is elevation of the eye; this is greatest when the eye is abducted. Secondarily, the muscle adducts and intorts the eye, these actions increasing as adduction increases.

Inferior Oblique Muscle

This muscle arises from the periosteum of the floor of the orbit, temporal to the lower portion of the lacrimal fossa. It passes laterally and posteriorly between the inferior rectus muscle and the floor of the orbit, being held in close approximation to the former by filamentary attachments and Lockwood's ligament. The insertion is variable; but, in general, the muscle inserts into the sclera beneath the lower portion of the lateral rectus muscle, behind the equator of the eye, and in a nearly horizontal plane beginning about 10 mm posterior to and slightly above the lower margin of the lateral rectus insertion; the inferior oblique insertion extends obliquely backward to within 4 or 5 mm of the optic nerve and the posterior ciliary vessels. The inferior temporal vortex vein exits approximately 6 to 8 mm below the scleral attachment of this muscle and about midway in its path.

The actions of the inferior oblique muscle are to elevate the eye when it is adducted, to produce extorsion by rotation on the anteroposterior axis, and to aid in abduction on the vertical axis.

Superior Oblique Muscle

This muscle arises from a thickened area of periosteum above and medial to the common ring tendon. It passes anteriorly at the junction of the medial and superior walls of the orbital fossa, and just behind the orbital margin it becomes tendinous to pass through the pulley near the superior orbital margin. The tendon then is reflected posteriorly and temporally to pierce Tenon's capsule and to pass between the superior rectus muscle and the globe to insert into the sclera behind the equator. The insertion begins 4 to 5 mm posterior to the insertion of the superior rectus muscle and fans out approximately 5 mm posteriorly along the lateral border of the muscle, the posterior edge being about 5 mm from the optic nerve and immediately temporal to the exit of the superior temporal vortex vein from the sclera. In the primary position the oblique tendon is only 2 to 3 mm from the nasal attachment of the superior rectus muscle. When the eye is rotated downward for operation on the tendon, this separation increases; however, numerous filamentary attachments extend from the superior oblique tendon to the superior rectus muscle, where the former passes under the latter. Many filamentary attachments also exist between the tendon fibers and the sheath which prevent too great retraction of the fibers when tenotomy is performed.

The primary action is to depress the eye when it is adducted; secondarily, the muscle intorts the eye along the anteroposterior axis and abducts the eye along the vertical axis. The anterior half of the reflected tendon of the superior oblique muscle may have a greater intorsional function, and the posterior half may have a greater depressor function.

PART TWO

Surgical Procedures

General Considerations

Instruments

Instruments which we find most satisfactory are shown in Figure 5. They include four fixation forceps, two Bishop Harmen or similar toothed forceps, six muscle hooks (two large, two medium, and two small), one pointed caliper, one Knapp scissors, one suture scissors, one Berens or Castroviejo eye speculum, one No. 10 straight Castroviejo needle holder, and a No. 3 Bard Parker knife with a No. 15 blade. Two Dyer extraocular muscle clamps (American V. Mueller, no. RD 1095) are preferred (Fig. 6). Refer to the Appendix for details.

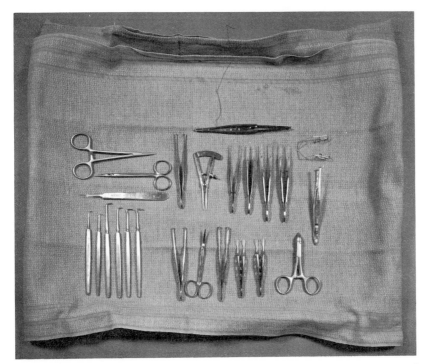

Figure 5. Instruments used in operations on eye muscles. (See text for description.)

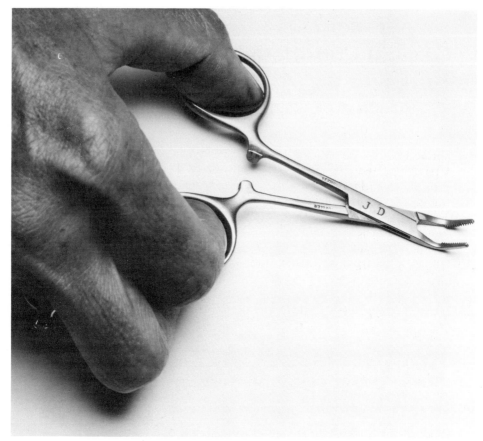

Figure 6. Dyer extraocular muscle clamp.

In addition, we use a Hildreth cautery to control excessive bleeding.

Suture Material

Absorbable Sutures. These are preferred for reattachment of muscles except in certain transposition operations.

1. Coated Vicryl (6-0) is our preference. It has good tensile strength and even caliber and is available in a 12-inch length with an S-24 Saberloc needle of the spatula type attached. This suture is retained for six weeks

and creates no postoperative reaction. Coated Vicryl (5-0) can be used when extra strength is needed for operating on patients with Graves' disease.

2. Plain collagen (6-0) with a G-1 micropoint cutting-type needle is ideal for conjunctival closure. It has sufficient tensile strength for this purpose and is available in 18-inch lengths. It is absorbed within seven to ten days.

Nonabsorbable Sutures.

Mersilene (5-0) with an S-24 Saberloc spatula-type needle is an excellent permanent suture that causes virtually no tissue reaction. It is used primarily for muscle-transposition procedures and for muscle or tendon tucks where permanence is desired. It is best to bury the knots and the ends of the suture under or in muscle, since the white color can be seen through the conjunctiva at times. Supramid Extra is another nonabsorbable suture that can be used; however, it has a few undesirable qualities. The cut ends of this suture must be heated by cautery in order to prevent conjunctival penetration by the sharp ends and lid irritation.

Preoperative Preparation

The patient's hair is covered with a scrub cap and the eyelids, nose, cheeks, and forehead are scrubbed with povidone-iodine (Betadine surgical scrub). Tincture of iodine may be applied to the bases of the lashes and eyebrows and rinsed away with sterile water. This last procedure is more necessary for intraocular than for muscle operations.

Drape the patient with sterile towels, a sheet, or plastic drapes, permitting only the eyes to be exposed.

Preparation of the eyes includes application of a 1:2500 solution of bichloride of mercury, a saline rinse, and instillation of phenylephrine 2.5 per cent. Adrenalin should not be instilled when halothane anesthetic is used. Apply a sterile eye drape to the operative side.

Postoperative Treatment

Immediate

1. Apply an antibiotic ointment, such as Blephamide, to the operated eye after closure of the conjunctiva.

2. Use no patch unless the operation involves cutting of two or more muscles of the same eye; then apply patch only to the operated eye. Even in

such circumstances, a patch often is applied only when the patient is an adult.

3. Ambulate patient as soon as possible.

After 24 Hours

1. Remove patch, if any, and cleanse eyes.
2. Allow infants or children to return home, but require that they return to be checked within seven to ten days.
3. Permit use of eyes to patient tolerance.
4. Prescribe no eye medications for children. Occasionally antibiotic-steroid drops, three times daily for a week to ten days, will be prescribed for adults.
5. Dismiss adults if they feel well enough.

Delayed

1. If eye is healing well after several days at the time of check, stop drops; prescribe as before if reaction is moderate to severe.
2. If suture reaction occurs after ten days to four weeks, treat with hot packs and steroid drops for three to four days.
3. Reexamine the patient at periodic intervals until all reaction subsides and the position of the eyes is stable.

Descriptions of Procedures

All diagrams (Figs. 7 through 21) are drawn from the surgeon's position at the head of the patient for the particular eye designated. The superior part of the illustrations are located inferiorly on the patient. Proximal, as used here, means toward the apex of the orbit; distal means toward the muscle insertion or the cornea.

Basic Incision of Conjunctiva and Tenon's Capsule Applicable to All Rectus Muscle Exposures

Exposure of the left medial rectus muscle is illustrated in Figure 7.

1. Figure 7A. Place traction suture adjacent to and about 1 mm from the limbus, securing both the conjunctiva and Tenon's capsule. Retract the globe away from the intended incision and grasp the conjunctiva with tissue forceps. Elevate the tissue and incise it 1 to 2 mm vertically with scissors about 1 to 2 mm posterior to the traction suture. Note plane of intended incision (Fig. 7A) which is completed after releasing the conjunctiva. The conjunctival incision should parallel the limbus and extend sufficiently far to be certain that both muscle edges are cleared. The closer to the limbus the incision is made, the less bleeding one encounters, and Tenon's capsule and the conjunctiva are conjoined near the limbus.

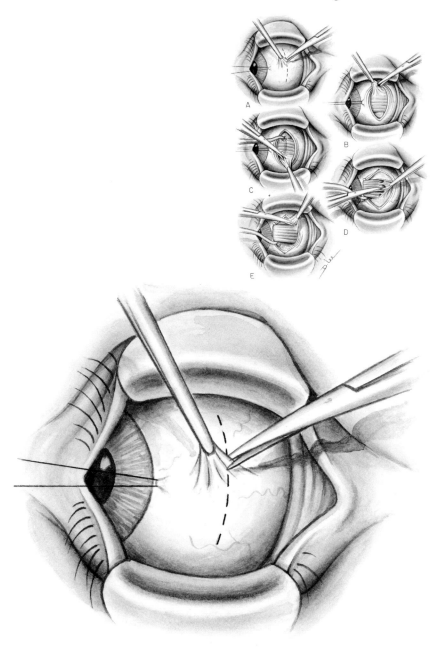

A

Figure 7. Basic incision of conjunctiva and Tenon's capsule, muscle exposure (left eye).   *Illustration continues*

23

2. Figure 7B. Pick up Tenon's capsule with tissue or toothed forceps well above or below the muscle plane and incise it with scissors, pointing the blades *away* from the muscle to avoid bleeding, which is brisk when the muscle is injured. Incise the capsule completely until bare sclera is noted, and spread the aperture with the scissors blades. Often several fine layers of Tenon's capsule appear to intervene. If difficulty is encountered in piercing the capsule, release the tissue and grasp each ensuing portion for complete incision. Any remaining tissue will hinder smooth passage of the muscle hook beneath the muscle.

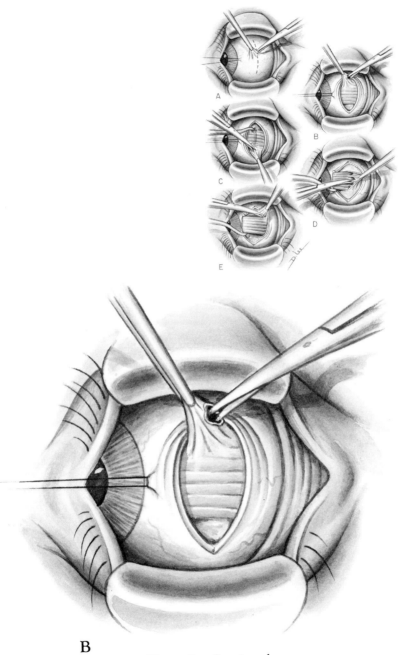

B

Figure 7. Continued.

Illustration continues

3. Figure 7C. Insert a medium-sized muscle hook through the aperture in Tenon's capsule and beneath the muscle, and tent the capsule upward on the opposite side of the muscle by rotating the tip of the hook. If the hook does not slide easily beneath the muscle, withdraw and reinsert it, keeping the hook point *flush* with the sclera. If the hook is passed too far posteriorly, other tissue may become engaged and distort the anatomy. Make a counterpuncture through Tenon's capsule beside the point of the hook, incising *away* from the muscle with scissors points. There is a tendency always to incise toward the muscle, but this usually results in muscle damage and bleeding since the entire muscle may not have been isolated. Once sclera is reached on the counterincision, slide a large hook beneath the muscle to exit at the original capsular incision. The entire muscle then should be secured.

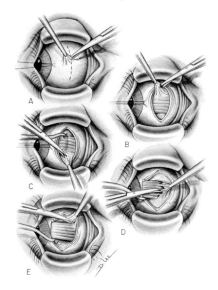

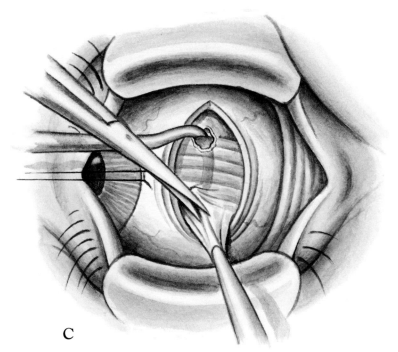

C

Figure 7. Continued.

Illustration continues

27

4. Figure 7D. Remove the traction suture and retract the globe with the muscle hook. Then, with forceps, pick up the conjunctiva and Tenon's capsule over the central part of the muscle and release the check ligaments and capsular tissue from the outer surface of the muscle, leaving a thin layer of muscle sheath intact over the fibers if possible. Avoid cutting through Tenon's capsule in order to prevent herniation of orbital fat into the operative site. Sever the check ligaments and adhesions as far posteriorly as possible to prevent retraction of tissues when the globe rotates in the direction of the operated muscle postoperatively; this is especially important in operations on the medial rectus muscle in order to prevent retraction of the caruncle on adduction.

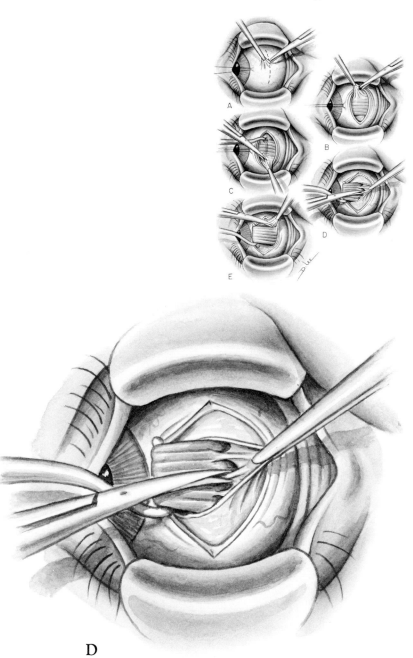

D

Figure 7. Continued.

Illustration continues

29

5. Figure 7E. Free the capsular tissue along both borders of the muscle as far posteriorly as feasible. Grasping the membranous material with forceps and rotating the globe in the opposite direction readily exposes the line of dissection. Caution should be exercised in freeing the lower border of the lateral rectus muscle and both borders of the superior rectus muscle to prevent, in the first instance, severing of the inferior oblique muscle as it passes beneath the lateral muscle to insert into the sclera or, in the second instance, injuring the superior oblique muscle as it courses beneath the superior rectus muscle.

If these basic principles are adhered to closely, muscle exposure is simple and free from complications. Remember to incise the conjunctiva relatively near the limbus and sufficiently far above and below the muscle and to buttonhole Tenon's capsule well above and below the muscle edges, cutting *away* from the muscle always.

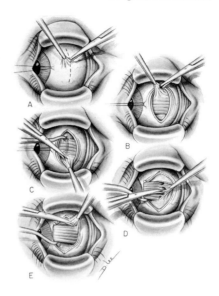

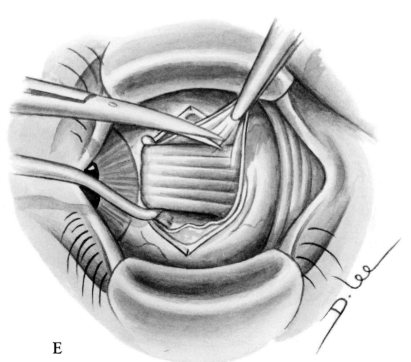

E

Figure 7. Continued.

Closure of the Conjunctiva and Tenon's Capsule

Since both layers were incised together, they are closed simultaneously. Eradicate all bleeding points before closing to prevent undue postoperative scarring.

1. Figure 8A. Pick up both layers at one extremity of the incision and close by means of a running mattress suture of plain collagen (6-0). This provides a smooth line for healing and little scar remains.

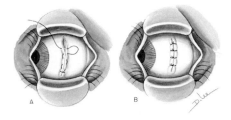

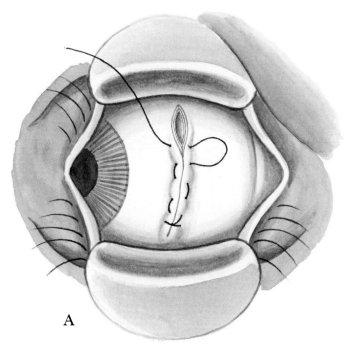

A

Figure 8. Closure of conjunctiva and Tenon's capsule (left eye).

Illustration continues

2. Figure 8B. Interrupted sutures of a similar material may be used, but they tend to pucker the tissues and are more likely to permit herniation of capsular tissue through the incision, which if incarcerated may result in cyst formation later. To prevent this, isolate the conjunctival edge carefully, closing it rather than Tenon's capsule alone.

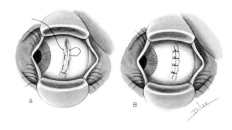

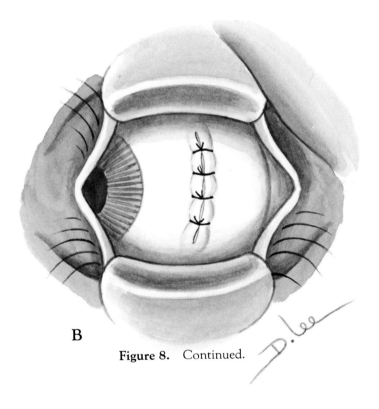

B

Figure 8. Continued.

Recession of Rectus Muscle

The procedure is essentially the same for each muscle.

1. Expose the muscle as described at the beginning of this chapter and as illustrated in Figure 7.
2. Figure 9A. Insert double-armed coated Vicryl (6-0) suture through the muscle substance to include the central one third and the entire thickness. Place the suture near the hook but allow room to sever the muscle between the suture and the hook. Tie a square knot and pass one arm of the suture *through* the muscle substance from the region of the knot to the edge. (Do not cut suture with needle.) Engage the lateral one third or one fourth of the entire muscle thickness with the suture and lock it securely. Follow the same procedure at the opposite edge and tighten the lock stitches by stretching both suture arms firmly.

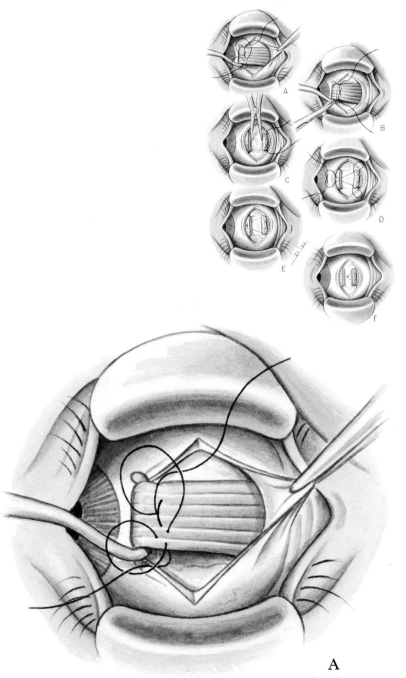

Figure 9. Recession of medial rectus muscle (left eye).

Illustration continues

3. Figure 9B. Retract the suture arms away from the muscle insertion and detach the muscle with scissors, cutting against the hook to prevent inadvertent penetration of the sclera and to leave a sufficient insertion remnant to identify the original site of insertion for topography now and during future operations. A small ridge does not show through the tissues postoperatively. (To ensure reattachment in the proper plane, some surgeons prefer to mark the sclera along the muscle edges with methylene blue or with a suture before they detach the muscle.) Permit the muscle to retract after ascertaining which suture arm is proper for each muscle edge to maintain orientation. The habit of leaving one end shorter for identification is good.

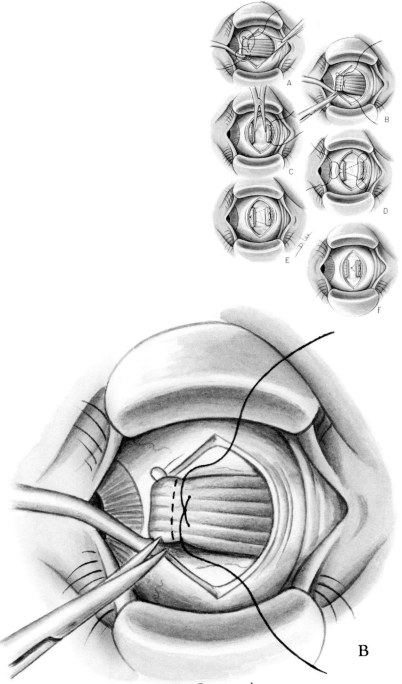

Figure 9. Continued.

Illustration continues

4. Figure 9C. Grasp the line of original insertion at one edge with tissue forceps, retract the globe to expose the sclera, and mark the desired distance of recession with calipers at both edges of the muscle. Avoid excessive pressure with the sharp points, especially at the area of original insertion, since perforation of the globe is possible. The arms of the calipers should extend from the point of previous insertion to the point at which the needle is to enter the sclera for reattachment, thereby giving an *exact* distance each time the procedure is performed.

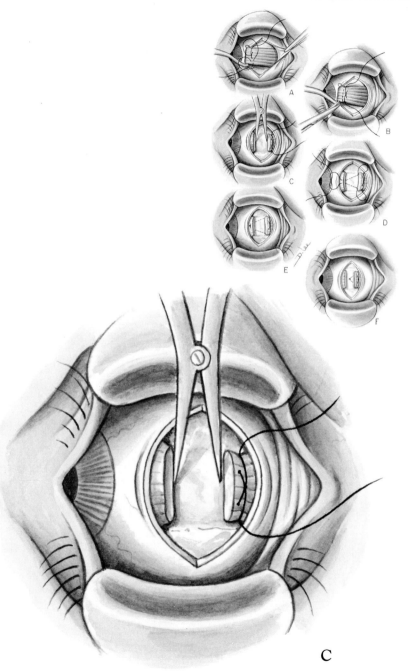

C

Figure 9. Continued.

Illustration continues

5. Figure 9D and E. Insert each needle in turn at the scleral mark and direct the needle toward the insertion at an angle approximating 45 degrees. The needle should be passed through the scleral substance (so that it is barely visible beneath the surface) for 1 to 2 mm before an exit is made. The needles also may be passed at 90 degrees to the intended line of insertion, but this has proved more difficult and less satisfactory

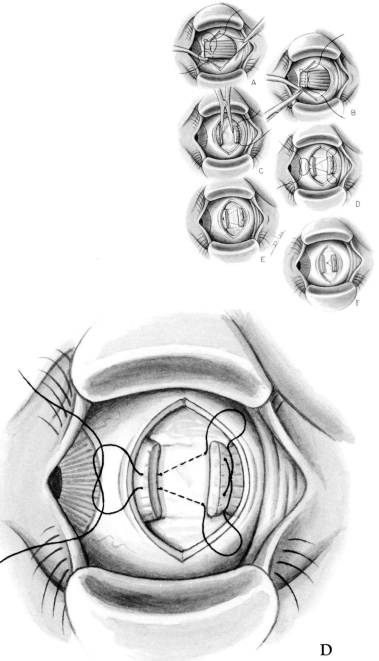

Figure 9. Continued.

D

Illustration continues

43

in our hands. Two modes of attachment are very satisfactory: (1) Figure
9D shows that both suture arms have been passed closely together
through the original insertion stump and have been tied as in Figure 9E.
This permits a secure attachment without undue stress on the suture,
but it leaves additional suture material in the operative site. (2) Figure

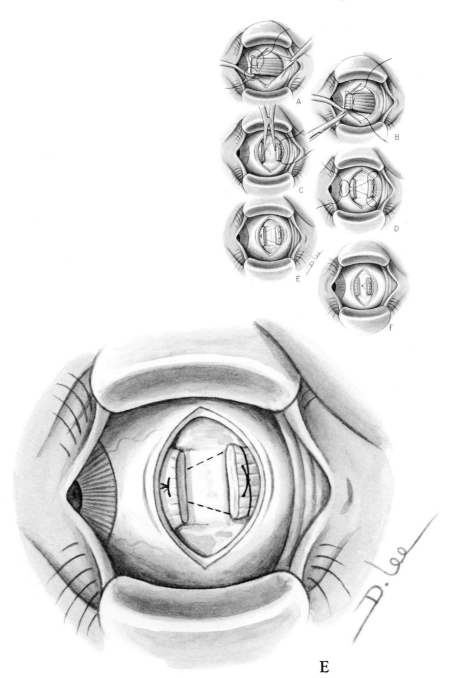

E

Figure 9. Continued.

Illustration continues

9F shows the sutures tied at the scleral exit site. A surgeon's knot is suggested to prevent inadvertent retraction of the muscle. These methods of reattachment prevent overriding of the intended future insertion by the muscle edge. An *exact* recession is the result. When recessing the superior and inferior rectus muscles, the angle of reattachment of the muscle to the globe should be the same (23°) as the original angle of insertion.

If a muscle clamp is used for recession operations, the sutures are inserted into the muscle proximal to the clamp in the manner just described, the muscle having been separated from the scleral insertion before suturing. Additional recession is required to allow for the 2 or 3 mm of tissue remaining distal to the suture when the clamp is released, since this tissue will override the point of entrance of the sutures and reduce the effectiveness of the recession.

6. Close Tenon's capsule and the conjunctiva as previously described (Fig. 8).

Adjustable Sutures. For patients with restrictive muscle problems, such as those from Graves' ophthalmopathy, multiple procedures, and paretic or paralytic conditions such as lateral rectus muscle palsy, some surgeons suggest the use of adjustable sutures.

In these situations, the double-armed suture is passed through the original insertion site with no other scleral bites. The muscle is permitted to retract until the surgeon believes it is an adequate or more than adequate recession. The suture is tied in a bow or ship knot so that it can be released. Usually, a supramaximal recession is done so that the muscle may be advanced hours later or the first day after surgery. Recessing a muscle is much more difficult.

Most surgeons who use the technique will admit that readjustment is not simple and, in most instances, not necessary because if one uses appropriate judgment at the time of the initial surgery, adjustment is not required.

In our experience, if one adjusts muscles until the pupillary light reflexes from the operating room light are the same in both eyes, the result in most instances is satisfactory.

In restrictive conditions, the position of the eye changes days to weeks after surgery so that an adjustment a few hours postoperatively may not remain as such.

The surgeon may think that a recession of 10 mm or more is achieved when, in fact, as the globe is released and arrives at its resting position, the relaxed muscle may creep forward several millimeters, and the intended recession is thus reduced.

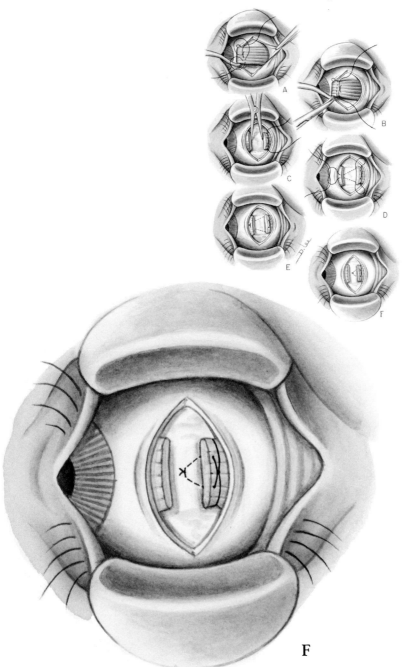

Figure 9. Continued.

47

The recession of a muscle more than one believes is actually necessary in order to adjust it later is, in our opinion, poor judgment.

Recession of Rectus Muscle with Displacement. The medial, superior, and inferior rectus muscles are used to illustrate these modifications.

1. Figure 10A and B. If the surgeon desires to move the rectus muscles downward, upward, or laterally for an "A" or "V" pattern, a similar technique is followed. Reattachment of the muscle to the sclera should be parallel to the plane of the limbus. Always allow 1 mm of recession for any detached rectus muscle, if it is to be reattached without an intended amount of recession, since some muscle tissue always is lost during suturing and reattachment. Failure to adhere to this point often will result in postoperative *overaction* of the muscle involved.

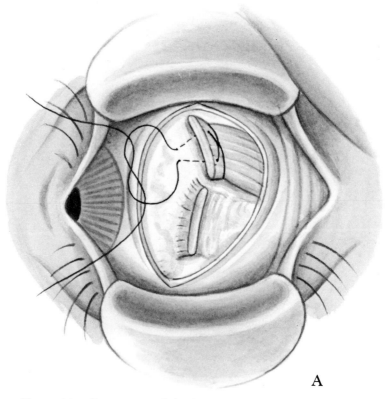

A

Figure 10. Recession and displacement of rectus muscle (left eye).

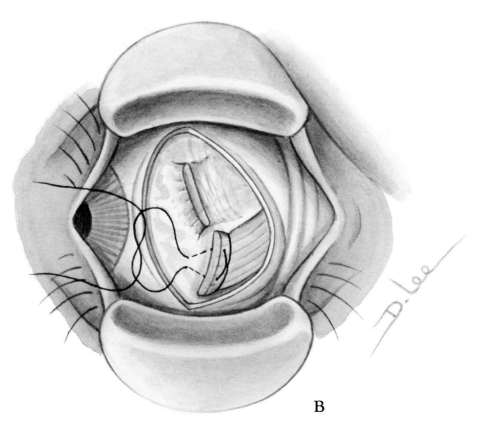

Figure 10. Continued.

2. Figure 11. *A* and *B* show recession of the superior rectus muscle.

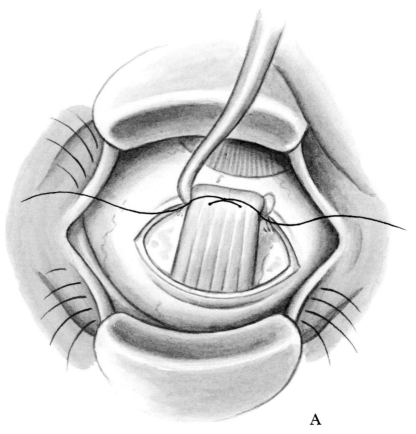

A

Figure 11. Recession and transposition of superior rectus muscle (left eye).

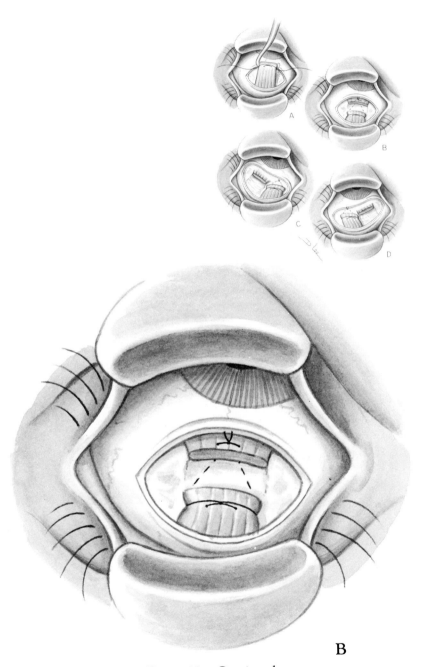

Figure 11. Continued.

B

Illustration continues

3. Figure 11. *C* and *D* illustrate moving the same muscle nasally and temporally to facilitate correction of a "V" or "A" pattern as noted in the preceding paragraph.

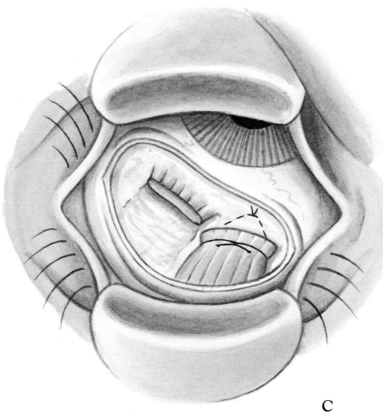

C

Figure 11. Continued.

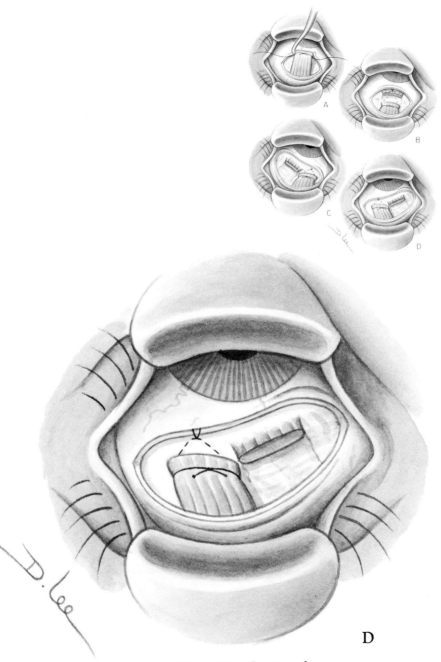

D

Figure 11. Continued.

4. Figure 12. *A, B, C,* and *D* illustrate similar procedures for the inferior rectus muscle.

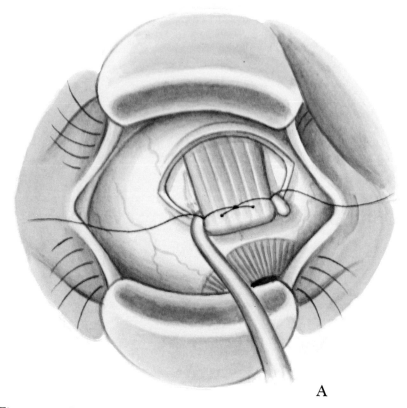

A

Figure 12. Recession and horizontal transplantation of inferior rectus muscle (left eye).

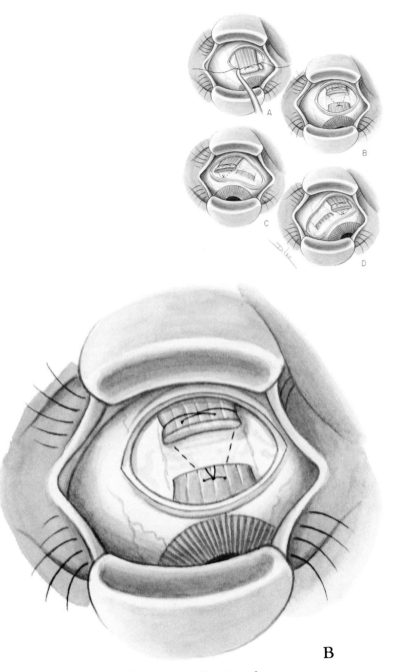

B

Figure 12. Continued.

Illustration continues

55

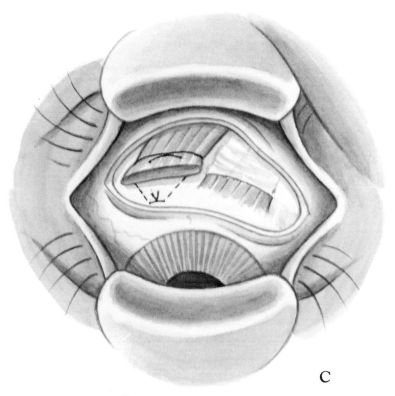

Figure 12. Continued.

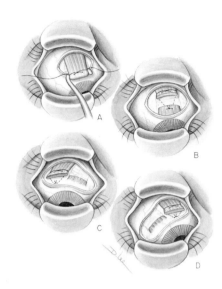

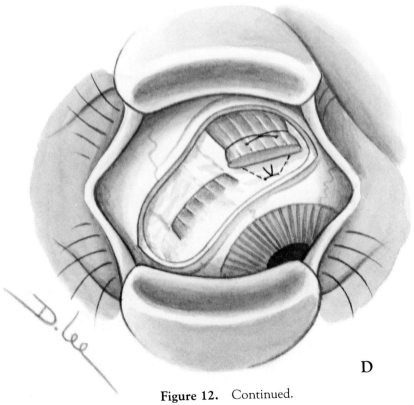

D

Figure 12. Continued.

Resection of Rectus Muscle

This procedure generally is the same for each muscle. Operation on the right medial rectus muscle is illustrated.

1. Expose the muscle as previously indicated (Fig. 7).
2. Figure 13A. Rotate the globe away from the site of resection and measure desired amount of resection with calipers. To attain reasonably repeatable results, measure from the top of the hook (at the insertion) to the point of intended placement of the sutures into the muscle. Naturally, the degree of tension on the muscle determines the amount of effective resection to some extent. Insert a second hook proximal to the desired suture site and insert suture as in Figure 13A.

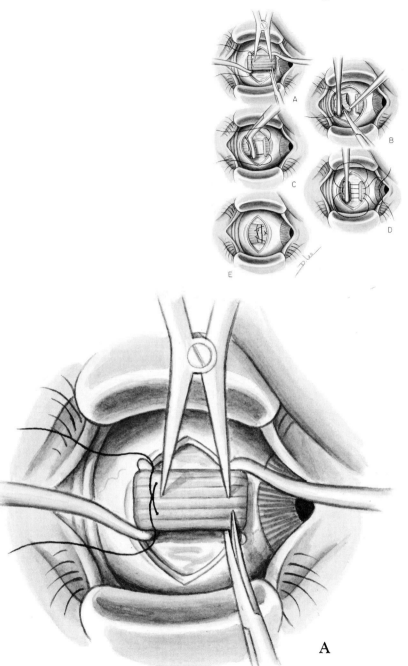

Figure 13. Resection of medial rectus muscle (right eye).

Illustration continues

3. Figure 13B. Apply muscle clamp just distal to the suture and sever the muscle near its insertion (Figs. 13A and B) with scissors, using the anterior hook as a "cutting board" to prevent penetration of the sclera and to leave a sufficient stump for reattachment of the muscle. Resect the muscle distal to the clamp. Often it is wise to leave the resection until all sutures are placed, as in Figure 13D, to prevent "losing" the muscle in the event that the clamp holds poorly, since recovery is thereby facilitated. Always retract the suture arms away from the site of intended resection.

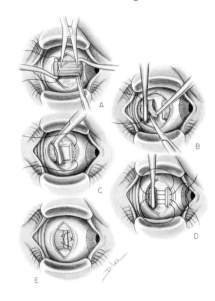

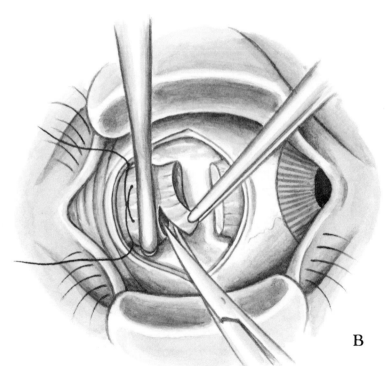

B

Figure 13. Continued.

Illustration continues

4. Figure 13C. To reattach the resected muscle, pass each suture through the insertion stump at either extremity and sufficiently into the substance of the sclera so that a "solid" hold is assured. Remember that the sclera is very thin at the point of muscle insertion, and penetration of the globe is possible if one is not diligent.

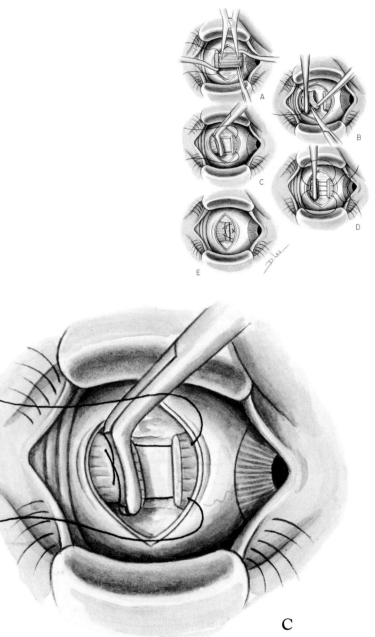

Figure 13. Continued.

Illustration continues

5. Figure 13D. Each suture arm is then carried back and through the central portion of the muscle just behind the original suture attachment and forward through the center of the insertion stump. This mode of attachment is secure and "slip-free," and it permits excellent approximation of the tissues.

An alternative method: Each suture arm is then inserted through the central portion of the insertion stump with a solid scleral "bite" and carried back through the central portion of the muscle just behind the original suture attachment and tied with a surgeon's knot.

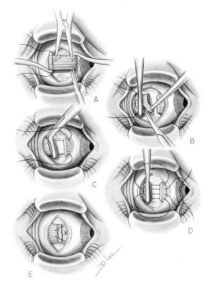

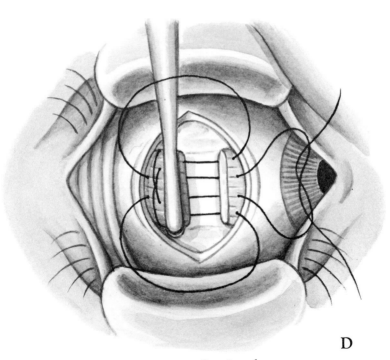

D

Figure 13. Continued.

Illustration continues

6. Figure 13E. The clamp is removed and the suture tied.
7. Close the conjunctiva and Tenon's capsule in the routine manner (Fig. 8).

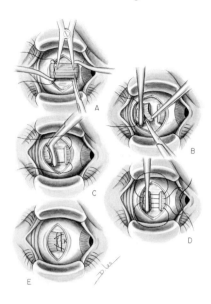

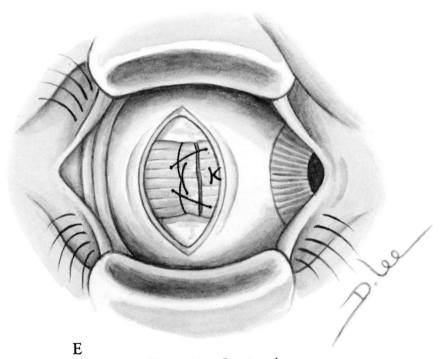

E

Figure 13. Continued.

Marginal Myotomy

The right medial rectus muscle is used to illustrate this effective secondary procedure.

1. Incise the conjunctiva and Tenon's capsule and isolate the muscle (Fig. 7).
2. Figure 14A. Retract the globe away from the desired operative site and apply a hemostat to include about one half the width of the muscle at its insertion. Ligate a portion of the muscle (at least one half of the muscle width) proximal to the clamp with absorbable suture to assure hemostasis, and remove the clamp.

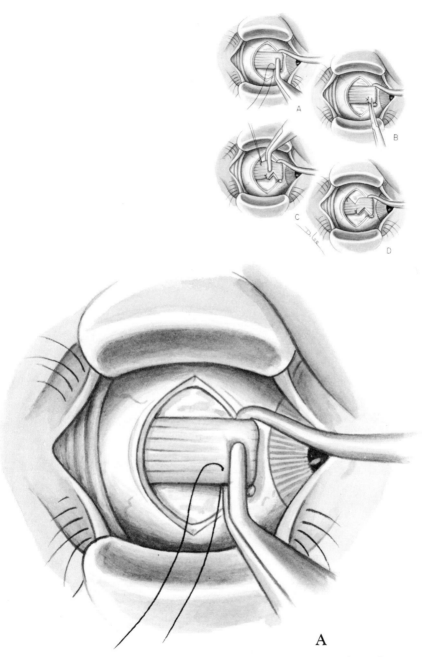

Figure 14. Marginal myotomy of rectus muscle (right eye).

Illustration continues

3. Figure 14B. With scissors sever muscle at least one half the width of the muscle.

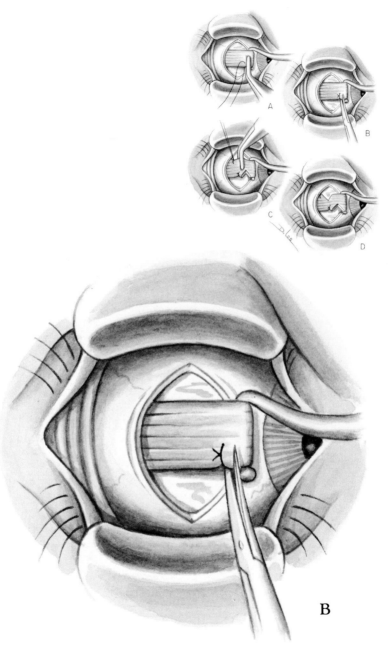

B

Figure 14. Continued.

Illustration continues

71

4. Figure 14C. Repeat the same procedure on the opposite side of the muscle and several millimeters proximal to the previous line of separation.

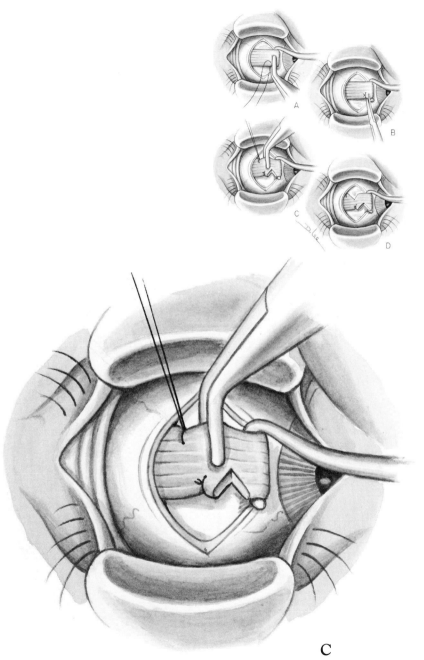

Figure 14. Continued.

C

Illustration continues

   5. Figure 14*D*. Sever muscle as in *B*.
   6. Close conjunctiva and Tenon's capsule in routine manner (Fig. 8).

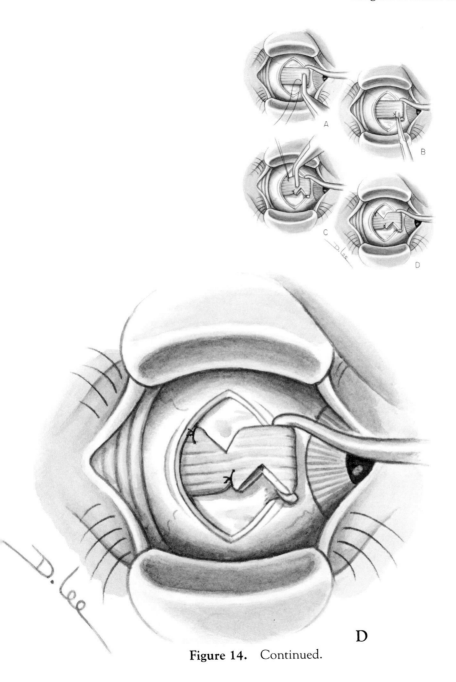

D

Figure 14. Continued.

Weakening the Inferior Oblique Muscle (Tenotomy or Disinsertion and Recession)

1. Figure 15A. Retract the globe upward and inward with a traction suture or forceps. Incise the conjunctiva and Tenon's capsule horizontally in the lower temporal quadrant of the globe so that the line of incision is covered by the eyelid postoperatively.

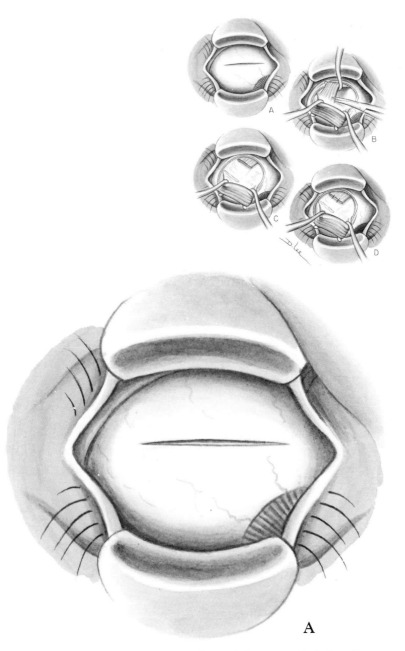

Figure 15. Weakening inferior oblique muscle (left eye).

Illustration continues

2. Figure 15B. Insert a muscle hook under the lateral rectus muscle insertion and maintain the globe in up-and-in position. Slide a medium hook between the lateral and inferior rectus muscles for about 10 mm, keeping the tip against the sclera and directed downward and backward (handle toward the operator). Turn the point of the hook upward (toward Tenon's capsule) and draw the inferior oblique muscle out of the incision. Direct the hook handle downward and outward and insert a second hook under the lateral muscle to expose the oblique insertion. The insertion is defined more accurately by bringing the closed scissors upward along the sclera until resistance of the insertion is met. Sever the tendinous portion of the muscle, flush with the sclera, along its entire attachment until the muscle pulls free of the hook. If a greater effect is desired, one can resect several millimeters of the distal end of the muscle, which should then be cauterized or ligated for hemostasis.

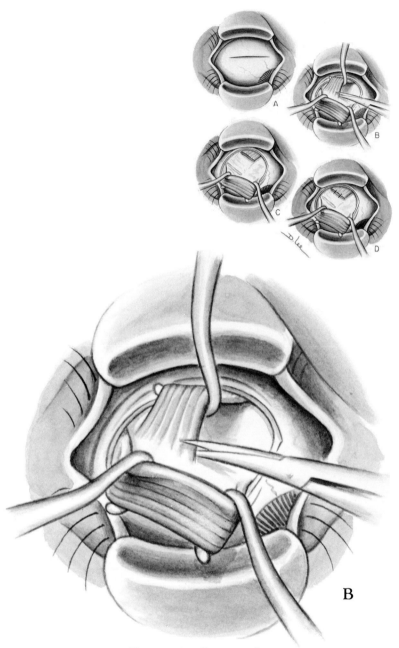

Figure 15. Continued.

Illustration continues

3. Figure 15C. Let the muscle retract into the wound without suturing.

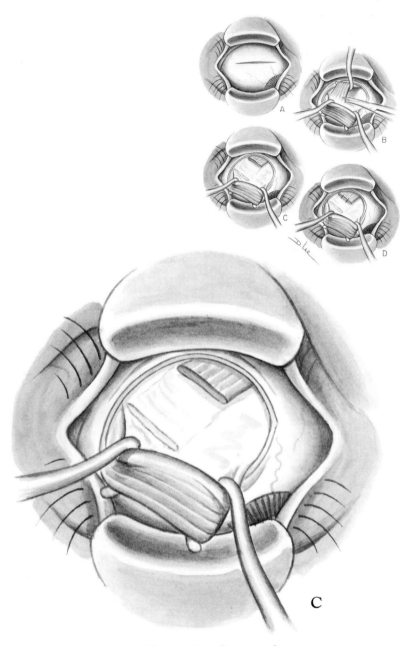

Figure 15. Continued.

Illustration continues

4. Figure 15D. An alternative method is to place sutures at the anterior and posterior borders of the muscle near its insertion. Free the muscle as in B, measure the desired amount of recession, and suture the muscle to the sclera as close to its original plane of attachment as possible. The amount of recession can be adjusted to the degree of inferior oblique muscle overaction: 6 mm recession for 1+ overaction, 10 mm recession for 2+ overaction, and 14 mm recession for 3+ overaction. Parks and Parker reattach the anterior corner of the inferior oblique 2 mm lateral and 3 mm posterior to the lateral border of the inferior rectus insertion. The posterior scleral reattachment is placed according to the width of the inferior oblique muscle.

5. Close the conjunctiva and Tenon's capsule in the routine manner (Fig. 8).

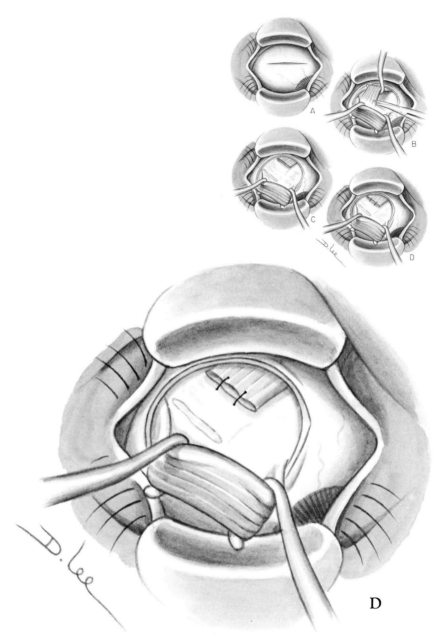

Figure 15. Continued.

Weakening the Superior Oblique Muscle

Various degrees of weakening may be achieved by intrasheath tenotomy, controlled tenectomy, and sheathotomy (Figs. 16C, D, and E, respectively).

1. Incise the conjunctiva and Tenon's capsule over the superior rectus muscle in the routine manner (Fig. 7) and expose muscle.
2. Figure 16A. Isolate the superior rectus muscle on a hook and rotate the globe downward and outward. Slide the tip of a medium hook along the sclera between the pulley and the medial border of the superior rectus muscle and backward 8 to 10 mm, turn the point upward toward Tenon's capsule, and draw the hook forward to engage the oblique tendon. Normally the tendon lies only a few millimeters behind the rectus insertion, but it slips farther back as the globe is rotated downward. Excess tissue often is engaged on the hook in addition to the tendon, but the glistening sheath usually is identified and isolated with relative ease. If many attempts are made without successful isolation, let the globe retract upward, slide the hook point under the rectus muscle in a down and back manner, and pull the hook nasally to engage the tendon.

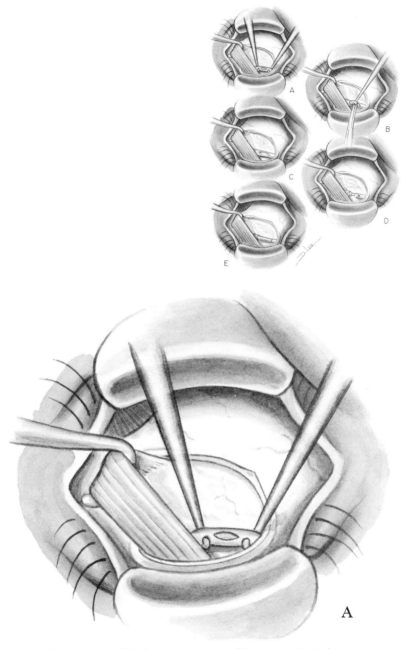

Figure 16. Weakening superior oblique muscle (left eye).

Illustration continues

3. Figure 16B. Once isolated, the tendon sheath is incised horizontally with a knife. The tendon fibers are isolated by teasing them out of the sheath with small hooks. They are then severed with scissors. This permits a portion of the sheath to remain intact. A tenotomy closer to the trochlea produces a greater weakening effect than one adjacent to the medial border of the superior rectus muscle.

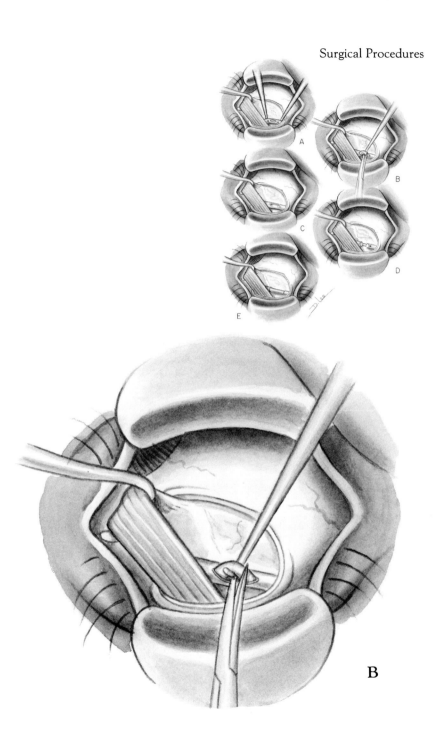

Figure 16. Continued.

Illustration continues

87

4. Figure 16C. This shows how the ends of the severed tendon fibers retract within the sheath after intrasheath tenotomy. Only a moderate degree of retraction of fibers is possible because of the numerous filamentary attachments of the tendon to its sheath. Retention of only small portions of the sheath seems adequate to allow function of the muscle postoperatively.

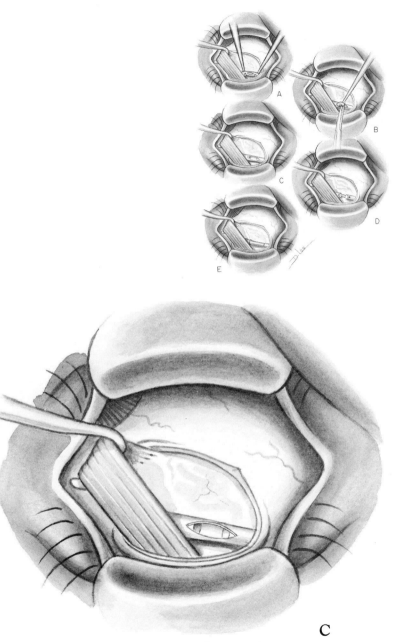

Figure 16. Continued.

Illustration continues

5. Figure 16D. An alternative procedure is controlled tenectomy: Isolate the tendon, place a mattress suture of nonabsorbable material, sever the tendon and sheath completely, and tie the suture to permit the degree of separation desired (usually 4 or 5 mm).

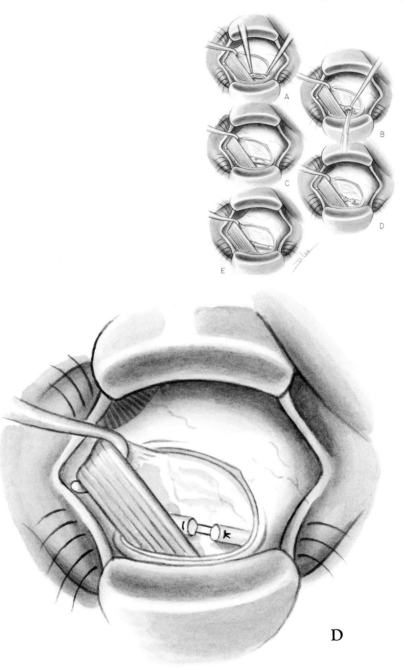

Figure 16. Continued.

Illustration continues

6. Figure 16E. If a weakening procedure involving only the sheath itself is desired, sheathotomy may be performed: The tendon is isolated as before, and the sheath is stripped from the tendon fibers from its point of exit from the capsular tissue near the pulley to the border of the rectus muscle, a distance of several millimeters.

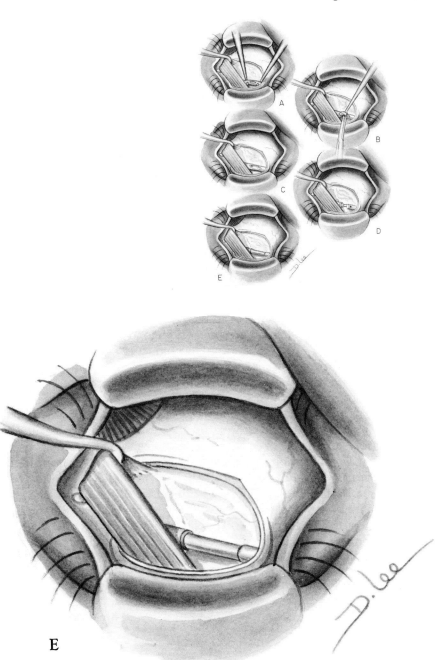

E

Figure 16. Continued.

Illustration continues

7. Close the conjunctiva and Tenon's capsule in the routine fashion (Fig. 8).

8. Figure 16F. An alternative method for doing a tenectomy of the superior oblique muscle is to use the temporal approach. The tendon is located 4 to 5 mm posterior to the lateral corner of the insertion of the superior rectus muscle and along the lateral border of the superior rectus muscle. Isolate the superior rectus muscle on a hook and rotate the globe downward and inward. *Carefully* search for the insertion of the superior oblique tendon. Its insertional fibers fan out as it fuses with the sclera at right angles to the lateral border of the superior rectus muscle. Engage the superior oblique tendon with a medium muscle hook and bring it temporally. Use scissors to carefully dissect the tendon free from the intermuscular membranes and the muscle capsule under the superior rectus muscle. The tenectomy can then be performed. A tenectomy closer to the trochlea has a greater weakening effect. Hooking and dissecting the tendon from the temporal side of the superior rectus muscle is associated with possible complications such as laceration of the vortex vein and inadvertent disinsertion of the tendon.

This procedure, when done with care, is the most effective and permanent for weakening the tendon without overcorrection.

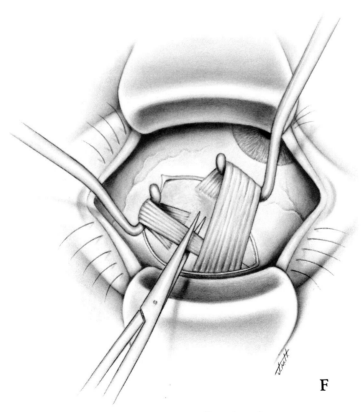

F

Figure 16. Continued.

Strengthening the Inferior Oblique Muscle

This can be achieved by means of tuck or advancement.

1. Figure 17A. Expose and isolate the inferior oblique muscle as described previously (Figs. 15A and B). The belly of the muscle temporal to the inferior rectus muscle is surrounded by much membranous material which must be stripped away gently to expose the muscle proper for 10 to 12 mm.

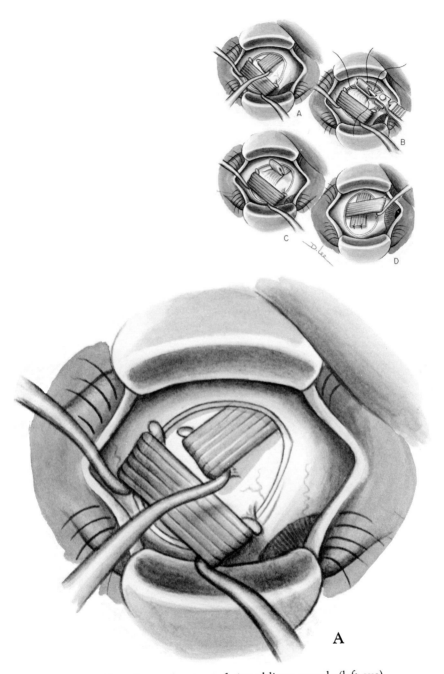

Figure 17. Strengthening inferior oblique muscle (left eye).

Illustration continues

2. Figure 17B. Insert a Fink tendon tucker, or simply tent the muscle upward, and obtain the desired amount of tuck (average about 8 mm total). Measure with calipers on each side of the tucker to find proper amount.

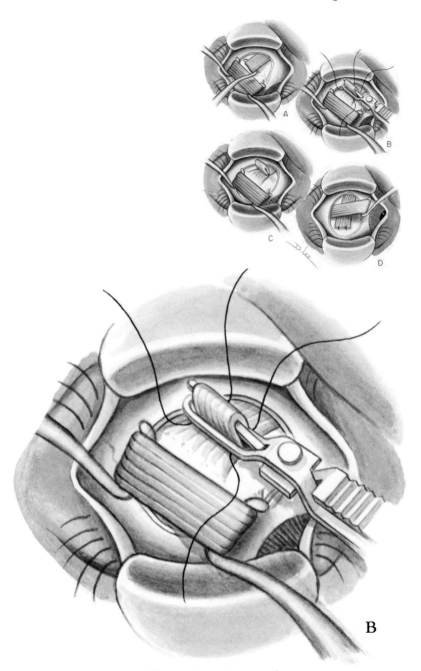

Figure 17. Continued.

Illustration continues

3. Figure 17C. Secure tuck by suturing at both *edges* of the muscle with nonabsorbable material. Place the sutures *beneath* the tucker blade (B). Include *only* the *outer one third* of the muscle in the sutures to prevent strangulation of the tissue.

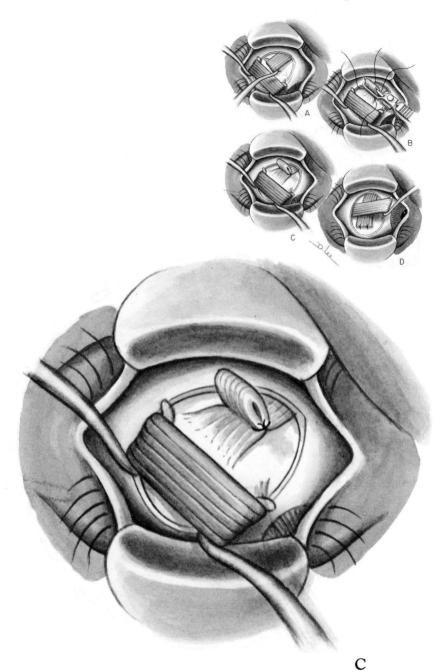

Figure 17. Continued.

C

Illustration continues

4. Figure 17D. An alternative procedure and one designed to give a somewhat more effective result is to advance the inferior oblique muscle upward beneath the lateral rectus muscle. The lateral rectus muscle is exposed in the routine fashion (Fig. 7). The inferior oblique muscle is isolated and sutures are placed as for a recession (Fig. 15), and the muscle is freed from the sclera. The lateral rectus muscle is elevated, and the oblique muscle is drawn upward beneath it to be sutured to the sclera slightly above (2 to 4 mm) the upper margin of the lateral rectus and in a plane approximating that of its normal insertion; that is, about 10 mm posterior to the attachment of the lateral rectus muscle.
5. Close the conjunctiva and Tenon's capsule in the routine manner (Fig. 8).

These strengthening procedures of the inferior oblique muscle are rarely indicated and are the least effective of the surgical procedures on the vertically acting muscles.

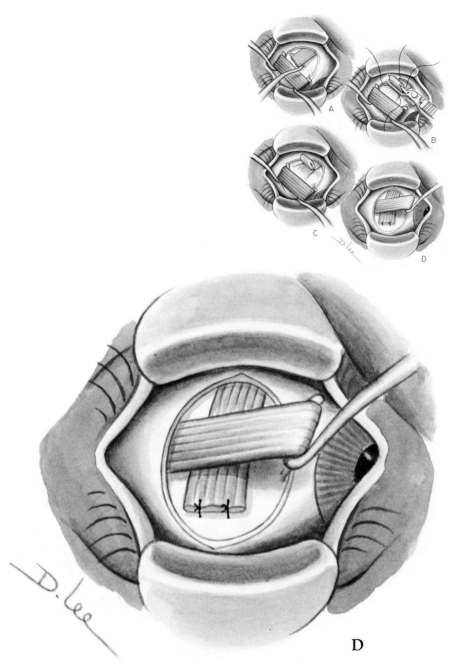

Figure 17. Continued.

103

Strengthening the Superior Oblique Muscle (Tuck)

1. Incise the conjunctiva and Tenon's capsule and expose the muscle in the routine manner (Fig. 7).

2. Figure 18A. Place a muscle hook under the superior rectus muscle near its insertion and rotate the globe *downward* and *inward*. Slip a medium hook, point against sclera, under the superior rectus muscle just behind its insertion and pass it backward and then temporally in a sweeping motion to secure the superior oblique near its insertion. Gently separate the filamentary attachments between the oblique muscle and the rectus muscle in order to draw the tendon laterally.

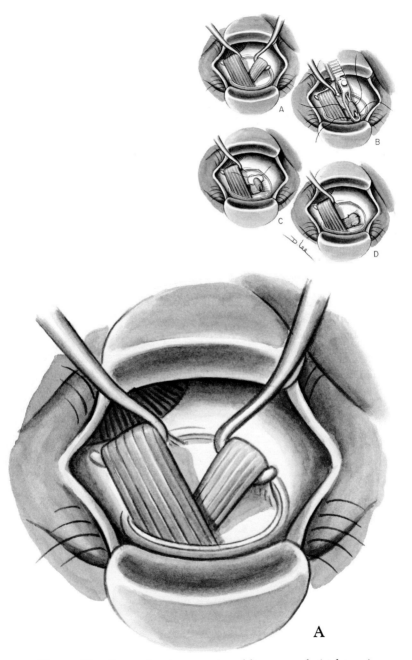

Figure 18. Strengthening superior oblique muscle (right eye).

Illustration continues

3. Figures 18B and C. Apply a Fink tendon tucker to secure the desired degree of tuck (about 4 to 5 mm on each side of the tucker arm for a total of 8 to 10 mm) and suture each edge with nonabsorbable material below the instrument. Avoid strangulating the entire tendon.

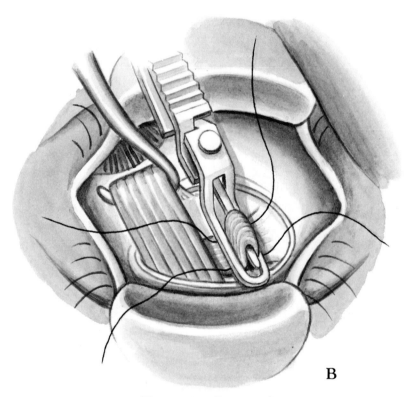

B

Figure 18. Continued.

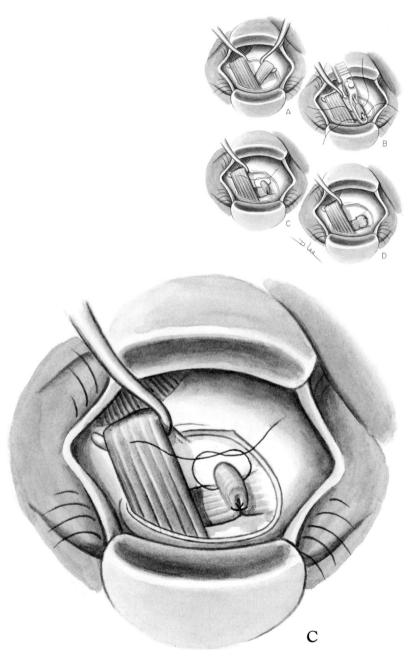

Figure 18. Continued.

Illustration continues

4. Figure 18D. Attach the tuck to the sclera near the insertion and in the same plane of attachment to avoid impingement of the tuck under the rectus muscle and to assure a permanent effect.
5. Close Tenon's capsule and the conjunctiva routinely (Fig. 8).

Alternative procedures include resection or temporal advancement of the entire tendon, but these are more difficult and less accurate.

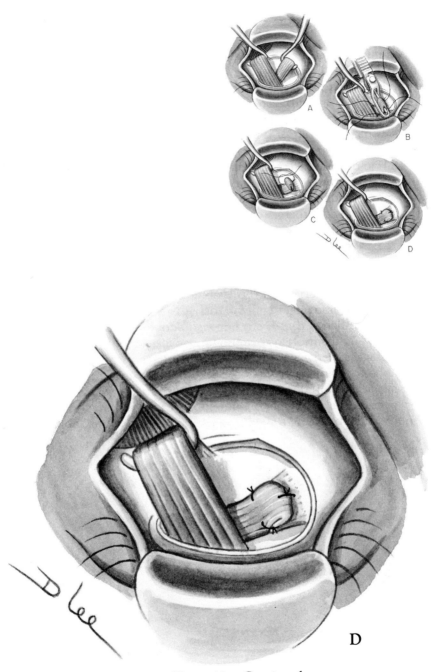

Figure 18. Continued.

Illustration continues

6. Figure 18E. A method to increase the intorsion function of the superior oblique muscle is the Harada-Ito procedure. In this procedure, the anterior half of the superior oblique tendon insertion is moved along the equator of the globe toward the superior border of the lateral rectus muscle. The insertion of the superior oblique muscle is isolated temporal to the superior rectus muscle as described previously. Then the tendon is divided for 10 mm along its length from its insertion. The posterior half of the tendon is left undisturbed. A coated Vicryl (6-0) suture is preplaced at the insertion of the anterior tendon, and the anterior half is disinserted. This portion of the tendon is then attached 8 mm posterior to the lateral rectus muscle insertion within 4 mm of the superior border of the muscle.

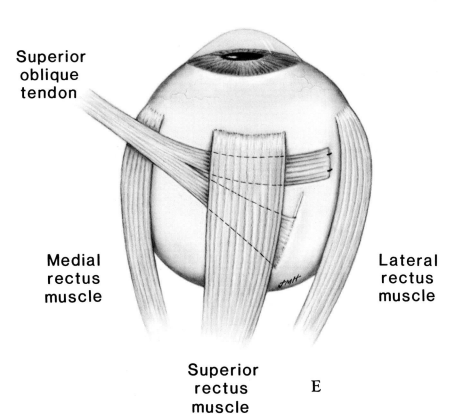

Superior oblique tendon

Medial rectus muscle

Lateral rectus muscle

Superior rectus muscle

E

Figure 18. Continued.

111

Muscle-Transposition Operations

Hummelsheim Procedure.   Operation on the right eye is illustrated in Figure 19.

1. Isolate and recess the antagonist to the paralytic muscle (the right medial rectus muscle in this instance) as previously described (Figs. 9, 10, 11, and 12).
2. Figure 19A. Expose and isolate the paralytic muscle (right lateral rectus muscle shown here) in the usual manner (Figs. 7 and 13) and resect the desired amount.

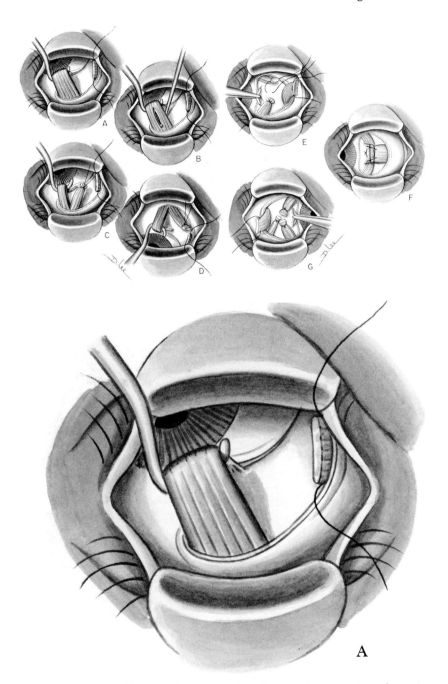

Figure 19. Hummelsheim procedure for muscle paralysis (right eye).

Illustration continues

113

3. Figure 19B. Permit the resected muscle to retract freely and continue the incision of Tenon's capsule and the conjunctiva around the globe to expose the superior and inferior rectus muscles in turn. Insert a hook under the superior rectus muscle, rotate the globe downward, and split the muscle with a small hook, taking about one half (or slightly less) of the muscle. Separate the fibers anteriorly to the insertion and posteriorly as far as possible.

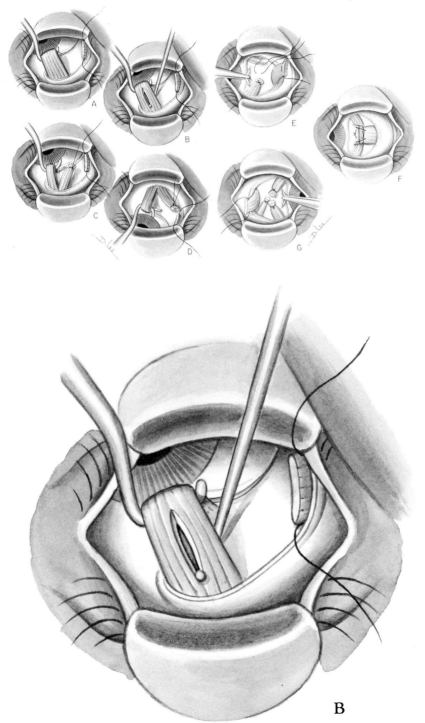

B

Figure 19. Continued. *Illustration continues*

4. Figure 19C. Place a suture (preferably nonabsorbable) at the distal end of the muscle slip and permit the muscle to relax freely.

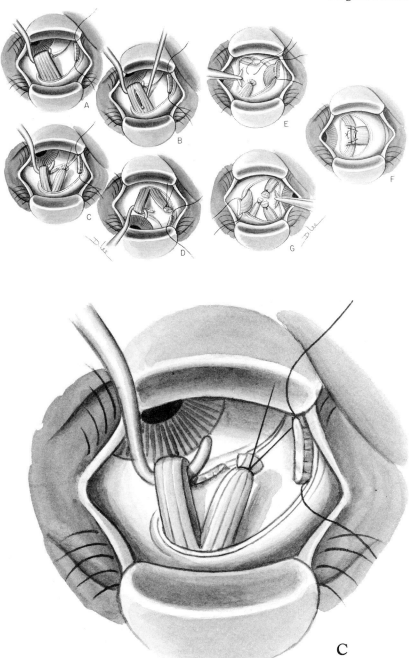

Figure 19. Continued.

Illustration continues

117

5. Figure 19D. Repeat the same procedure for the inferior rectus muscle.

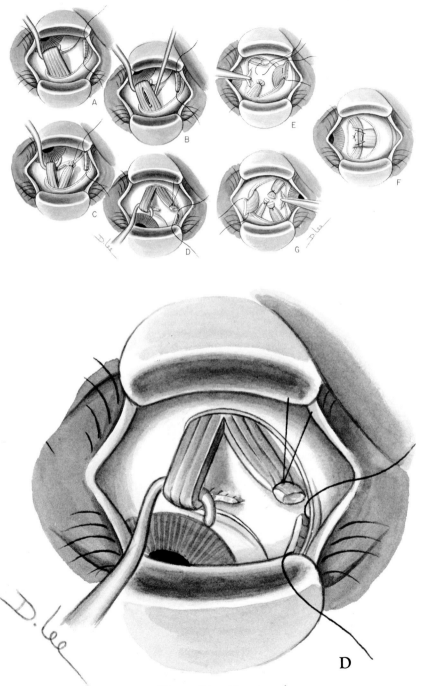

Figure 19. Continued.

Illustration continues

119

6. Figure 19E. Attach the superior and inferior muscle slips to the sclera just behind the insertion stump of the resected rectus muscle so that they nearly touch. Ideally they can be sutured together to increase the effectiveness of the operation.

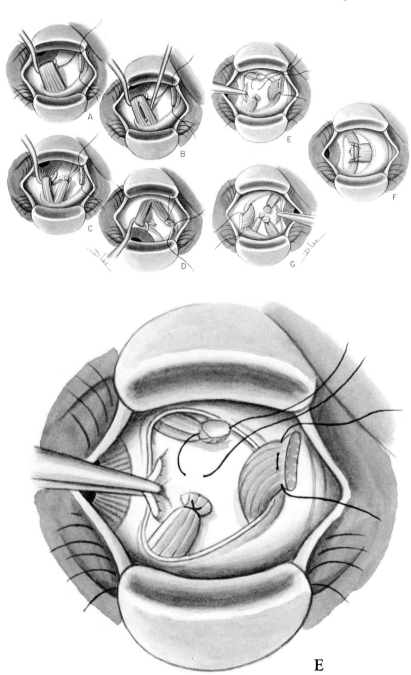

Figure 19. Continued.

E

Illustration continues

7. Figure 19F. Reattach the resected muscle to the original insertion in the manner illustrated (Fig. 13) so that it overlies the transposed muscle slips.

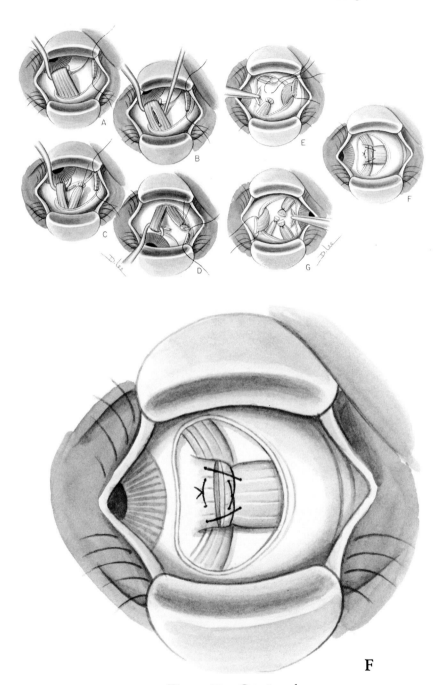

Figure 19. Continued.

F

Illustration continues

8. Figure 19G. This illustrates the transposition of the superior oblique tendon to the same position as the rectus slips for medial rectus paralysis. The oblique tendon is severed nasal to the superior rectus muscle and attached as shown to aid in fixation of the globe, especially in N-III paralysis. The resected rectus muscle (right medial rectus in the illustration) then is reattached at the original insertion.

9. Close the conjunctiva and Tenon's capsule for each exposure (Fig. 8).

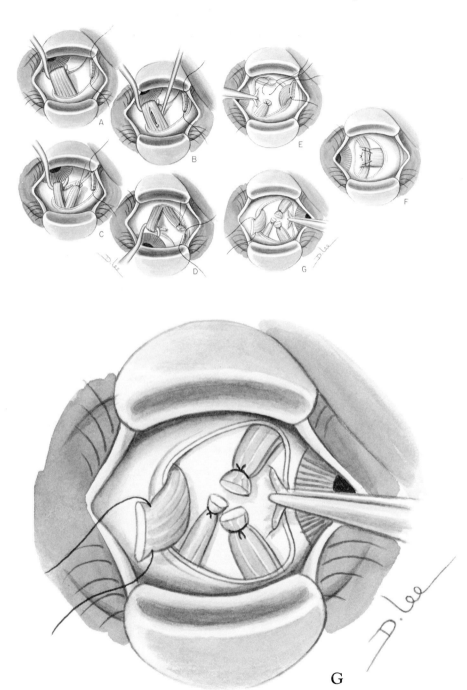

Figure 19. Continued.

125

Whole-Muscle Transposition for Muscle Paralysis (Left Eye Shown)

1. Figure 20A. Expose and recess the antagonist of the paralytic muscle.

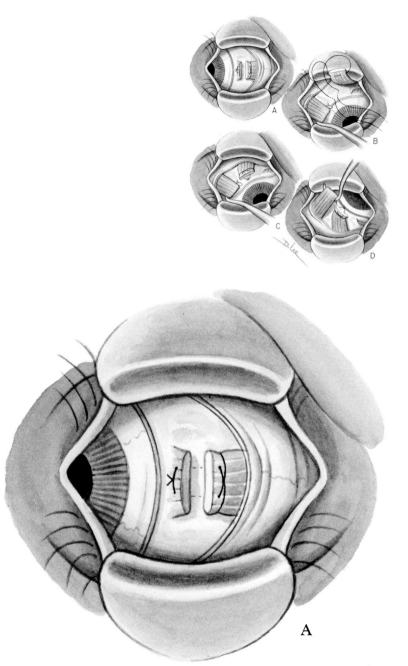

Figure 20. Whole-muscle transposition accompanying horizontal rectus muscle recession (left eye). *Illustration continues*

127

2. Figure 20B. Extend the incision to expose the inferior and superior rectus muscles as well as the paralyzed muscle. Isolate the inferior rectus muscle, place sutures, and detach the muscle from its insertion.

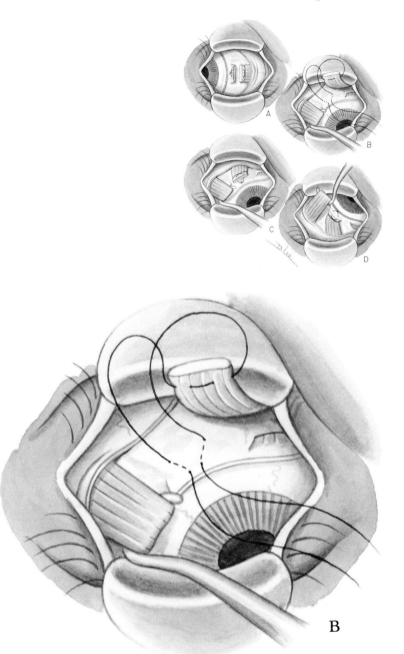

Figure 20. Continued.

Illustration continues

129

3. Figure 20C. Reattach the inferior rectus muscle to the sclera at the lower margin of the lateral rectus muscle, representing a nearly 90 degree transposition. Reattachment should be in the plane of the limbus.

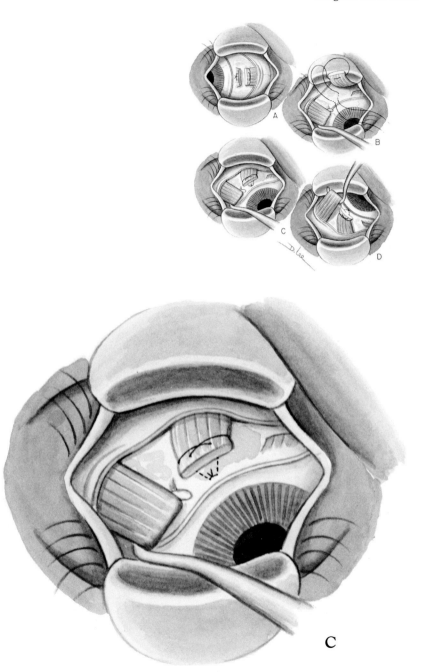

C

Figure 20. Continued.

Illustration continues

131

4. Figure 20D. Detach and transpose the superior rectus muscle in a similar manner.
5. The paralyzed lateral rectus muscle is left intact.
6. Close the incision in the usual manner (Fig. 8).

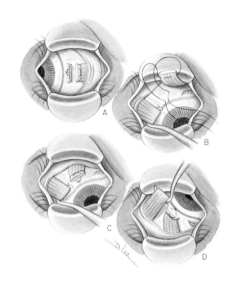

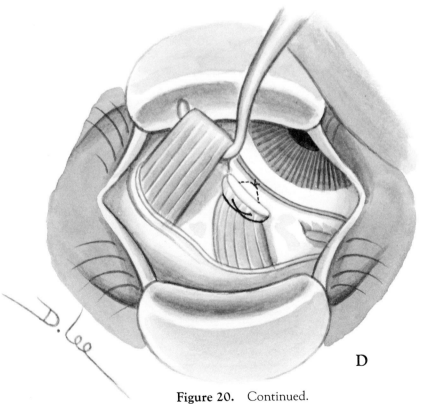

D

Figure 20. Continued.

Jensen Procedure

1. Isolate and recess the antagonist to the paralytic muscle (the medial rectus muscle in this instance) at least 7 to 8 mm.
2. Expose and isolate the paralytic muscle (lateral rectus muscle in this case) in the usual manner and split the muscle in half lengthwise with a small muscle hook. Separate the fibers anteriorly to the insertion and posteriorly as far as possible.
3. Expose and isolate the superior rectus and inferior rectus muscles and repeat the same procedure for each. Preserve the vessels in the nasal half of the muscles.
4. Tie the lateral half of the superior rectus muscle to the superior half of the lateral rectus muscle, and tie the lateral half of the inferior rectus muscle to the inferior half of the lateral rectus muscle with nonabsorbable sutures. A small scleral bite 15 mm from the limbus and midway between the two joining muscles may be taken with each suture in order to prevent the suture from slipping anteriorly (Fig. 21).
5. Finally, close the conjunctiva and Tenon's capsule for each exposure in the usual manner. The conjunctiva over the medial rectus muscle may be recessed.

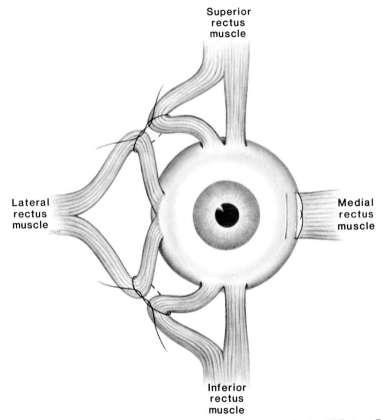

Figure 21. Jensen procedure. (From Lee, D. A., Dyer, J. A., O'Brien, P. C., and Taylor, J. Z.: Surgical treatment of lateral rectus muscle paralysis. Am. J. Ophthalmol. 97:511–518, 1984. By permission of Ophthalmic Publishing Company.)

135

PART THREE

Additional Considerations for Each Operation

Recession of Rectus Muscles

Medial Rectus Recession (Figs. 9 and 10)

The incision of the conjunctiva and Tenon's capsule of a child or young adult may be 2 or 3 mm from the limbus; but for older patients, because the tissues are much thinner and more friable, the incision should be several millimeters from the limbus and a traction suture should not be used. This applies to all procedures.

Clear the intermuscular membranes and Tenon's capsule as *far posteriorly* as possible to prevent retraction of the caruncle and semilunar fold on adduction.

For *children* less than 14 years old the *usual* recession is 5 mm. For *adults* 5.5 mm is adequate, except for paralytic strabismus (which will be described subsequently). As noted in the discussion of Figure 9C, the muscle "stops" at the point of entrance of the needle into the sclera; thus, an exact and repeatable recession can be made. The additional 0.5 mm allows for tissue "lost" in suturing and severing the muscle. *If greater amounts of recession are performed, weakness of adduction and convergence may result.*

In monocular procedures a maximal recession always is done.

For an "A" or "V" pattern the muscle is reattached in a position higher or lower on the globe, respectively, but always the new insertion should parallel the limbus. The muscle usually is moved its full width for effective results (Figs. 10A and B).

Lateral Rectus Recession

Clear Tenon's capsule and the intermuscular membranes as *far posteriorly* as possible, but exercise *caution* at the lower edge; otherwise, the inferior oblique muscle may be cut inadvertently since many filamentary attachments exist between the muscles. When the lateral rectus muscle has been detached, elevate it posteriorly to free it from the sclera and the inferior oblique muscle.

139

A *maximal recession* is *6.5 mm* for *children* less than 14 years old and *7.5 mm* for *adults*, the 0.5 mm allowing for tissue lost in suturing and releasing the muscle. This permits reattachment to the sclera at the equator. *Greater amounts of recession weaken abduction*, as is occasionally needed in paralytic strabismus or multiple operations.

For an "A" or "V" pattern move the *entire muscle its full width* downward or upward, respectively, and reattach it to the sclera with the line of attachment parallel to the limbus. Lesser amounts of transposition usually do not effect the desired result.

Superior Rectus Recession (Fig. 11)

For exposure of this muscle remember that the nasal edge of the insertion is somewhat closer to the limbus than is the temporal edge, the insertion forming an angle of 23 degrees with the visual axis. Also, the superior oblique muscle is closer to the insertion of the superior rectus muscle nasally. Because of these relationships, the muscle hook usually should be passed from the temporal side, allowing one to engage the rectus muscle more easily and to prevent engaging the superior oblique tendon as well.

Free the intermuscular membranes and Tenon's capsule as far posteriorly as possible, using care not to sever the levator above and the superior oblique tendon on either side. Filamentary attachments occur between the oblique and rectus muscles, and these should be severed gently before recessing or moving either muscle.

A *maximal recession* is *4.5 mm* for patients of any age. *Greater amounts may result in retraction of the upper eyelid and weakness of elevation;* and lesser amounts, except for release of the muscle for detachment surgery or muscle transposition, are seldom indicated. Remember to recess the additional 0.5 mm to compensate for loss of tissue during suturing. In fact, one should recess this small amount, or even 1 mm, if the muscle is detached for another operation only. If it is not recessed, postoperative overaction may result.

For "A" or "V" patterns move the muscle temporally or nasally the *full width* for an effective result. *Nasal placement aids convergence; temporal placement aids divergence.*

Inferior Rectus Recession (Fig. 12)

Expose and clear the muscle as for other recession procedures but avoid too deep a penetration of Lockwood's ligament and injury to the inferior oblique muscle which underlies it. Usually no difficulty is encountered; but, for difficult recessions—as frequently found in cases of ophthalmopathy of Graves' disease—one needs to dissect the rectus muscle as free as possible from the underlying oblique muscle to effect an adequate recession and reattachment.

A *recession of 4.5 mm* usually is *maximal* for patients of all age groups to prevent retraction of the lower eyelid or a weakness of depression of the globe postoperatively. However, a recession greater than this (up to 5 or 6 mm) may be necessary in Graves' ophthalmopathy because the contracted muscle cannot be placed closer to the limbus.

For an "A" or "V" pattern the muscle is moved nasally or temporally its *full width* and recessed 1.0 mm to effect an adequate result and to prevent postoperative overaction as noted previously. The new line of insertion should parallel the limbus. *Nasal placement aids convergence while temporal placement aids divergence.*

Marginal Myotomy of the Rectus Muscle

Marginal myotomy (Fig. 14) usually is used as a *secondary* lengthening or weakening procedure. It will give an *effective lengthening* of the muscle of 2 to 3 mm. It is very useful when a rectus muscle previously has been recessed a maximal amount and a slightly greater weakening is desired, especially if the manipulation of severing and resuturing the muscle is undesirable. Also, when a *previously resected muscle* needs to have its action reduced only slightly, myotomy is successful.

As a primary procedure it is useful only if minimal weakening is desired.

Tenotomy

Inferior Oblique Tenotomy (Disinsertion) (Fig. 15)

A lower quadrant incision gives adequate exposure for tenotomy and permits healing with minimal scarring. Also, the scar is not apparent in this position.

The globe should be rotated well up and in, and the inferior oblique muscle should be secured as described in the discussion of Figure 15B. The tip of the hook should be kept in contact with the sclera and pointed upward as it is moved under the oblique muscle. Then the tip should be pointed outward to secure the muscle and pull it nasally and upward out of the incision.

Identify the insertion carefully with the closed scissors and release the muscle flush with the sclera by means of short snips with the scissors until the muscle slips freely off the hook. At times the membranous tissue joining the oblique and lateral rectus muscles must be separated before the oblique muscle is freed completely.

If one cannot identify easily the most posterior tip of the insertion to release it, it is better to sever the taut muscle fibers which remain and then stop any bleeding rather than chance injury to the posterior ciliary arteries.

After tenotomy let the muscle retract into the surgical site. No bleeding should occur if only the tendinous condensation has been cut at the insertion. If bleeding occurs or persists, tie or cauterize the bleeding points before closing.

In closing Tenon's capsule and the conjunctiva, elevate them well to be certain that the oblique muscle has not been included in the closure.

Our experience with inferior oblique tenotomy is discussed in the Appendix.

Superior Oblique Surgery (Fig. 16)

The incision should be made over the nasal edge of the superior rectus insertion and carried more nasally to expose the operative site

143

since the nasal border of the superior rectus, being near the limbus, is easily secured for this procedure. Buttonhole Tenon's capsule well to the nasal side, and after the muscle is secured, enlarge the capsular incision nasally. The rectus muscle does not need to be exposed completely.

To secure the tendon of the oblique muscle between the pulley and the superior rectus pass a medium hook posteriorly for several millimeters with the tip pointed temporally and against the sclera. Then turn the tip upward and pull the hook forward. The tendon will appear as a shiny tube among much capsular tissue. Use small hooks to isolate it.

Once the tendon sheath has been incised, tease the fibers out of the sheath and sever them. At least a remnant of the sheath must remain to maintain the action of the superior oblique muscle.

A preferable and more effective procedure is a tenectomy of the superior oblique tendon temporal to the superior rectus muscle. The tendon is secured on a hook from beneath the superior rectus muscle and severed completely. The effect is greater when the tendon is severed closer to the superior rectus muscle. The filamentary attachments of the tendon to the superior rectus muscle prevent total weakening of the superior oblique muscle. Disinsertion and recession of the superior oblique muscle have been described, but we do not believe that they are as effective.

Resection of a Rectus Muscle

Medial Rectus Resection (Fig. 13)

Expose the muscle well back to permit easier application of sutures and clamps.

A resection of 6 to 7 mm may be made with reasonable ease. Greater amounts require much traction and thereby add to the difficulty of the procedure. However, up to 10 mm may be resected with effort. Usually it is preferable to resect the opposite medial muscle a moderate amount also.

Utmost care should be used to prevent suture breakage, since the muscle can be lost irretrievably if a large resection has been performed. Any major resections may result in relative enophthalmos and impaired rotation in the opposite direction.

Lateral Rectus Resection (Fig. 13)

Carry exposure of the muscle well back to free all of Tenon's capsule and the intermuscular membranes along its edges. Watch carefully for the inferior oblique insertion in order to avoid injuring it when freeing the lower border of the rectus muscle.

Before resecting the muscle lift it upward to separate any membranous attachments to the underlying inferior oblique muscle, which may be incorporated into the suture or clamp for the resection. In that event, when the rectus muscle is reattached to the sclera, an effective advancement or tucking of the oblique muscle may result.

Avoid resection of more than 10 or at most 11 mm to prevent retraction of the globe postoperatively with narrowing of the fissure and nonconcomitance of rotation (reduced adduction on the operated side).

After reattaching the muscle to the area of insertion, be certain that other tissues are free along the muscle edges and separate additional intermuscular membranes and Tenon's capsule, which have been exposed.

145

Superior Rectus Resection (Fig. 13)

When exposing the superior portion of the muscle, exercise care in severing Tenon's capsule and the intermuscular membranes. The levator may be traumatized if the separation is made too far posteriorly. Bleeding can occur but is infrequent.

As in the case of recession, guard against injuring the superior oblique muscle as it passes beneath the rectus muscle. Before resecting and reattaching the muscle, elevate it to be certain that the oblique muscle is not included in the suture or clamp and free any membranous attachments between the muscles.

A resection of greater than 4 mm may result in ptosis of the upper eyelid.

Clear all excess tissue from around the muscle if any has been included in suturing it to the site of insertion.

Conjunctival incisions heal more quickly when covered by the eyelids, and less postoperative swelling ensues.

Inferior Rectus Resection (Fig. 13)

As in the use of recession, exercise care to free all intermuscular membranes and Tenon's capsule as far posteriorly as possible, but avoid injury to the inferior oblique muscle passing beneath the inferior rectus muscle.

A resection of greater than 4 mm may result in ptosis of the lower eyelid.

After reattaching the rectus muscle, clear any excess tissue which may have become attached during resection or suturing. Also, free any additional Tenon's capsule and intermuscular membranes which may appear after the shortening procedure.

Our experience with bilateral medial rectus recession and lateral rectus resection for the treatment of congenital esotropia is discussed in the Appendix.

Tuck of Oblique Muscle

Inferior Oblique Tuck (Advancement) (Fig. 17)

A tuck rather than resection and reunion of the muscle is desired to avoid bleeding and to permit release of the tuck should it prove to be too great in degree. For this the Fink tendon tucker is a useful instrument. When fully opened it will result in a 10-mm shortening (5 mm on each side of the tucker blade). Usually about an 8-mm tuck is required for an effective result.

After securing the inferior oblique muscle between the inferior and lateral rectus muscles, free the capsular tissue to expose the muscle belly as much as possible so that a tuck can be made easily. Secure the tuck with nonabsorbable suture. Include only the outer third on each side to avoid strangulating the muscle completely.

Advancement of the muscle upward beneath the lateral rectus muscle may yield a greater effect; but this requires securing that muscle with sutures near its insertion, freeing the inferior oblique muscle at its insertion, exposing the lateral muscle so that the oblique muscle can be slid upward beneath it, and reattaching the oblique muscle to the sclera 2 or 3 mm above the upper border of the lateral rectus muscle and hopefully in a plane nearly approximating that of the original insertion. The described tuck seems to yield effective results and, being simpler, is recommended.

Superior Oblique Tuck (Fig. 18)

This relatively simple procedure increases the effective action of the muscle.

Free the intermuscular membranous union between the superior rectus and oblique muscles so that the superior oblique tendon may be drawn temporally with ease. Form the tuck on the temporal side always.

A graded tuck can be used, but if the defect is enough to require operation, a tuck of 8 to 10 mm usually is required.

Try to avoid surrounding the entire tendon with the securing suture; however, since tendon only is involved, little trouble is encountered if it does occur.

Use nonabsorbable suture and attach the tip of the tucked tendon to the sclera in the normal plane of muscle attachment.

The Harada-Ito procedure may be useful for the treatment of the torsional aspect of superior oblique palsy. It is usually performed bilaterally for bilateral superior oblique palsy in which a vertical component is absent but there is an increasing esotropia on downgaze as well as 7° to 20° of excyclotropia in primary gaze and more in midline downgaze. Bilateral advancement of the tendon to the superior border of the lateral rectus muscle corrects 15° to 20° of excyclodeviation, and the midline downgaze esotropia is also corrected with this procedure.

Muscle-Transposition Operations (Figs. 19, 20, and 21)

Do not detach all four rectus muscles at one operation since anterior segment ischemia and sector iris atrophy most likely will occur. If one half or even one third of a muscle (usually two muscles are involved) is left intact (as in a Hummelsheim procedure [Fig. 19]), an adequate blood supply to the anterior globe seems assured.

When transpositioning whole muscles (Fig. 20) (as for an "A" or "V" pattern) with no intent to have a recession also, be sure to reattach the muscles in a plane parallel to the limbus and recess at least 1 mm to avoid overaction of the muscle postoperatively. Move the muscle at least its full width for a positive effect.

Transposition of the whole superior and inferior rectus muscles should be to the upper and lower edges, respectively, of the paretic or paralytic muscle to be aided since, in our experience, a lesser transposition gives an ineffective result.

Recess the direct antagonist of the paretic muscle, but do *not* detach the paretic muscle (to prevent iris atrophy) if two other rectus muscles are to be detached.

The Jensen procedure (Fig. 21) may have a lesser chance of causing anterior segment ischemia than the Hummelsheim procedure or whole-muscle transposition because only one muscle is disinserted.

Our experience with the various surgical treatments for abducens muscle paralysis is discussed in the Appendix.

PART FOUR

Indications for and Types of Operative Procedures

We have found all procedures suggested in this book to be effective and safe. If they are performed according to the directions in the preceding pages, we think consistent results can be obtained.

Young muscle surgeons, and some older ones, often ask, "How much surgery must we do for this amount of deviation?" Usually the reply is that experience will help one to reach the correct answer. However, we believe that definite guidelines can be given, especially for uncomplicated cases, and that such rules-of-thumb can be effective. Surely one can do better than just operate and hope for the best.

We trust that those colleagues who frown on the formulation of specific instructions will agree after fair trial that these procedures are indeed about what they would do.

Although forced duction tests are useful, we rely chiefly on the values for deviation determined by cover tests in the cardinal positions and on versions and convergence. Correction of the defect as it "appears" gives adequate results; this holds, in general, for reoperations as well.

Convergent Strabismus

The following discussion and flowchart concern only convergent strabismus that persists after all means of nonsurgical treatment have been exhausted.

The treatment of esotropia (ET) is presented in the flowchart on pages 156–57. First, one must determine whether the ET varies with fixation on near or distant objects. If the ET is greater when the patient fixates on near objects, the amount of the accommodative component can be determined by observing how the ET changes with a full spectacle correction from a cycloplegic refraction. If this completely resolves the ET, then the ET is primarily accommodative and the treatment is a full spectacle correction or miotics. No surgery is indicated in accommodative ET unless there is residual ET even with the full cycloplegic spectacle correction. In this situation, surgery should be done to correct most of the ET without the spectacle correction, and the spectacle correction can be adjusted postoperatively. In those cases in which the ET is partially accommodative or nonaccommodative, one should check whether the patient has an "A" or "V" pattern.

If there is no "A" or "V" pattern, recess both medial rectus muscles (MR's) 5.5 mm for deviations up to 50 prism diopters (pd) in adults. For deviations greater than 50 pd, add a single lateral rectus muscle (LR) resection, preferably on the nondominant eye. Usually 5 mm is adequate. For deviations of 60 pd or greater, recess both MR's 5 mm and resect both LR's 5 mm for 50 pd of deviation, 6 mm for 60 pd, and 8 mm for 80 pd (maximum). If there is an "A" pattern ET with overactive superior oblique muscles, then both MR's should be recessed 5 mm and a tenectomy should be done of both superior oblique muscles. If there is no superior oblique overaction, both MR's should be recessed 5 mm and moved superiorly one muscle width. If this fails, then both superior rectus muscles should be moved temporally one muscle width. If there is a "V" pattern ET with overactive inferior oblique muscles, then both MR's should be recessed 5 mm and a disinsertion should be done of both inferior oblique muscles. If there is no inferior oblique overaction, both MR's should be recessed 5 mm and moved inferiorly one muscle width. If this fails, then both inferior rectus muscles should be moved temporally one muscle width. Very large esotropic deviations may necessitate the addition of LR resections to these procedures (as in the situation in which there is no "A" or "V" pattern).

If the ET is equal at near and far fixation, the MR's and LR's of one eye are operated on. Usually, this is done on the amblyopic or primarily deviating eye. The MR is recessed 5.5 mm and the LR is resected 4 mm for 20 pd of deviation, 6 mm for 30 pd of deviation, and 8 mm for 40 pd of deviation. If there is greater than 50 pd of ET, the other MR is recessed 5.5 mm.

If the ET is greater at distant fixation than at near fixation, the patient has a divergence insufficiency. The surgical treatment for this would be bilateral LR resections of 4 mm for 20 pd of deviation, 6 mm for 30 pd of deviation, and 8 mm for 40 pd of deviation. If there is greater than 50 pd of ET, one MR is recessed 5.5 mm. In adults, less surgery is required to achieve results comparable to those in children.

Equal Vision Alternators

Those patients who present a greater esodeviation for near fixation and who have a normal or excessive near point of convergence (NPC) (convergence excess type) with an ET should have an "innervational" type of procedure rather than a "mechanical" one.

Recession of Both Medial Rectus Muscles. Recess each MR 4 to 5 mm up to 30 pd of deviation plus 0.5 mm for loss of tissue due to suturing, to a maximum of 4.5 mm for patients 14 years old or younger and of 5.5 mm for those older than 14.

Examples:
1. For deviations up to 50 pd, recess each MR 5.5 mm.
2. For deviations greater than 50 pd, recess each MR 5 mm and add a single LR resection. This should be 5 mm.
3. For deviations of 60 pd or greater, recess each MR 5 mm and resect each LR 5 mm for 50 pd, 6 mm for 60 pd, and 8 mm for 80 pd.

(Refer to the chart, "Four Relatively Uncommon Strabismus Disorders," on pages 164–65.)

"A" Pattern Esotropia (Greater Esodeviation on Upward Gaze)

Patients in this group will have 15 to 20 pd greater ET on upward gaze than in the primary position; for example, a patient may have 0 deviation on downward gaze, 20 pd ET in the primary position, and 35 pd ET on looking up.

Recession of Both Medial Rectus Muscles. The first choice among corrective procedures is recession of both MR's an amount necessary to correct ET in the primary position *and* movement upward of both MR's an amount equal to the width of the muscles.

For the example just given, recess MR's 5 mm and move them upward one muscle width.

Temporal Placement of Superior Rectus Muscles. Second choice among procedures is placement of the superior rectus muscles (SR's) one *full muscle width* temporally to increase divergence on upward gaze. Probably this is best used as a secondary procedure, when the MR's have already been operated on and an "A" pattern ET persists or appears secondarily.

Strengthening of Inferior Oblique Muscles. This procedure is a possible third choice. Some surgeons think underaction of these muscles is responsible for the "A" effect. Either a tuck of 6 mm or more of each inferior oblique muscle (IO) or an advancement of the IO to the upper border of the corresponding LR is required to enhance the action. Use this procedure only if a definite underaction of the IO's can be demonstrated.

"V" Pattern Esotropia (Greater ET on Downward Gaze)

Patients in this group should have at least 15 pd greater ET when looking down than in primary position.

Recession of Both Medial Rectus Muscles. The procedure of choice for this problem is recession of MR's the amount necessary to correct ET in primary position and downward placement one muscle width.

Example: For 0 deviation on upward gaze, 20 pd ET in primary position, and 40 pd ET on downward gaze, recess MR's 5 mm and move down one muscle width.

TREATMENT OF ESOTROPIA

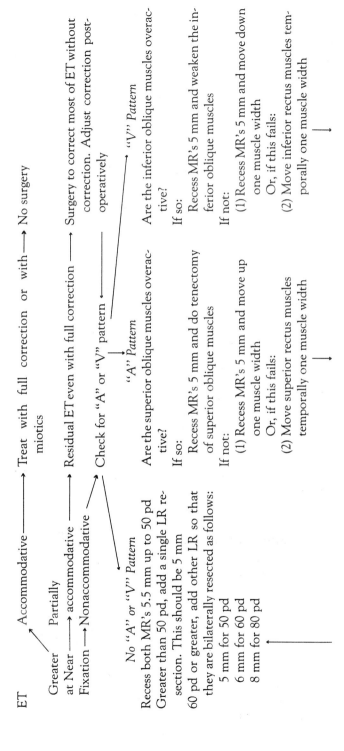

ET

Greater at Near Fixation → Accommodative → Treat with full correction or with → No surgery
miotics

Partially accommodative → Nonaccommodative → Residual ET even with full correction → Surgery to correct most of ET without correction. Adjust correction post-operatively

Check for "A" or "V" pattern

"A" Pattern

Are the superior oblique muscles overactive?

If so:
Recess MR's 5 mm and do tenectomy of superior oblique muscles

If not:
(1) Recess MR's 5 mm and move up one muscle width
Or, if this fails:
(2) Move superior rectus muscles temporally one muscle width

"V" Pattern

Are the inferior oblique muscles overactive?

If so:
Recess MR's 5 mm and weaken the inferior oblique muscles

If not:
(1) Recess MR's 5 mm and move down one muscle width
Or, if this fails:
(2) Move inferior rectus muscles temporally one muscle width

No "A" or "V" Pattern

Recess both MR's 5.5 mm up to 50 pd
Greater than 50 pd, add a single LR resection. This should be 5 mm
60 pd or greater, add other LR so that they are bilaterally resected as follows:
5 mm for 50 pd
6 mm for 60 pd
8 mm for 80 pd

Very large ET's may necessitate the addition of LR resections to these procedures (as is done when there is no "A" or "V" pattern)

ET Equal at Near and Far Fixation ——→ Recess MR and resect LR in one eye ——→ Recess MR 5.5 mm
Resect LR as follows:
4 mm for 20 pd
6 mm for 30 pd
8 mm for 40 pd
If greater than 50 pd, recess the other MR 5.5 mm

ET Greater at Distant Fixation ——→ Divergence Insufficiency ——→ Resect LR's as follows:
4 mm for 20 pd
6 mm for 30 pd
8 mm for 40 pd
If greater than 50 pd, recess one MR 5.5 mm

Operate on the amblyopic or primarily deviating eye as a general rule. In adults, less surgery is required to achieve results comparable to those in children.

Temporal Placement of Inferior Rectus Muscles One Muscle Width.

This second choice procedure to improve divergence on downward gaze is perhaps best used as a secondary operation when the MR's have been operated on previously and a "V" pattern persists or develops secondarily.

Strengthening Superior Oblique Muscles.

This third-choice procedure is used when evidence indicates a definite weakness of the superior oblique muscles (SO's). A tuck of 6 mm or more is usually required to produce an effective result.

Weakening Inferior Oblique Muscles.

If there is evidence of IO overaction, a weakening procedure such as tenectomy or tenotomy should be performed unilaterally or bilaterally.

Crossed-Fixation Pattern

In these cases the ET usually is present at birth in an amount of 40 pd or more. The patient fixes to the left with the right eye and to the right with the left eye, converges excessively, and abducts poorly to either side, although some LR action usually can be demonstrated on ductions. Vision is good in both eyes. Since abduction is poor, more than a bimedial recession is in order.

Recession-Resection Procedure.

An effective procedure for ET of 40 pd is a 5 mm recession of *both* MR's and a 5 mm resection of *one* LR, usually of the nondominant eye. For ET of 50 pd or greater, we recommend bilateral recession-resection procedures. A useful guide is to recess *both* MR's 5 mm for 50 pd and to resect *both* LR's 6 mm for 60 pd and an additional 1 mm for each 10 pd of ET to a maximum of 8 mm. If one or both IO's are overactive, they should be weakened at the same time, preferably bilaterally.

Example: For crossed fixation with 70 pd of ET, recess MR's 5 mm and resect LR's 7 mm.

(Refer to the Appendix for the treatment of severe congenital ET.)

Monocular Esotropia

If the deviation is the same for distant and near fixation, if one prefers a uniocular procedure to a binocular one, if the deviating eye is amblyopic, or if the operation is contemplated for cosmetic purposes primarily, a recession of one MR combined with resection of the ipsilateral

LR is in order. Some surgeons think operation on the dominant eye is more effective in correcting the ET, but operating on the nondominant eye if vision is equal in both eyes or on the convergent eye with amblyopia or other defect is usually quite satisfactory.

Recession-Resection Procedures

For ET of 20 pd or More. Recess one MR 4.5 mm for patients up to age 14 years or 5.5 mm for patients older than 14 years *and* resect one LR 1 mm/5 pd of deviation, starting at 4 mm for 20 pd. The recession is maximal in each instance; only the resection need vary and 10 mm is usually the upper limit, as noted early in the text.

Examples (patients less than 14 years old):

1. For deviation of 20 pd, recess MR 4.5 mm and resect LR 4 mm.
2. For 30 pd, recess MR 4.5 mm and resect LR 6 mm.
3. For 40 pd, recess MR 4.5 mm and resect LR 8 mm.
4. For 50 pd, recess MR 4.5 mm and resect LR 10 mm.
5. For more than 50 pd, recess both MR's 4.5 mm and resect LR 5 mm or more as deviation increases.

For ET Less Than 20 pd Which the Surgeon Feels Must Be Corrected. Recession of one MR 4.5 mm (for patients age 14 or younger) and resection of the ipsilateral LR 4 mm produce a lasting result with little chance of overcorrection. A single MR recession in our opinion is less effective since many patients have anomalous correspondence with this degree of deviation and their eyes will return to the old angle shortly after operation.

Comment. A recession-resection operation is preferred in all instances of ET when the NPC is remote.

Such an operation may be considered a "mechanical" one, since the eye in a sense actually is moved from one position to another.

Divergence Insufficiency

Patients with divergence insufficiency have greater esodeviation far than near; for example, such a patient may have an ET of 30 pd at distant fixation and of 10 pd at near fixation.

Lateral Rectus Resection. Resect both LR's 1 mm/5 pd of deviation, starting at 4 mm for each eye for 20 pd of ET. This corrects the far error without overcorrecting the near.

Examples:

1. For a deviation of 20 pd ET on far fixation, resect both LR's 4 mm.
2. For 30 pd ET far, resect both LR's 6 mm.
3. For 40 pd ET far, resect both LR's 8 mm.
4. For 50 pd ET and over, recess one MR 5 mm and apply rules given previously.

(Refer to the chart, "Four Relatively Uncommon Strabismus Disorders," on pages 164–65.)

Convergent Strabismus with Associated Vertical Anomalies

Usually these appear in the form of IO overaction in one or both eyes. At times there may be SO overaction, although this is much less frequent. Vertical rectus muscles are involved rarely.

Overaction of Inferior Oblique Muscles.
If the defect is monocular, do a tenotomy in conjunction with the operation for ET. Do not expect to influence ET greatly if tenotomy alone is done. If IO overaction is bilateral to any degree, do a bilateral tenotomy even if one IO is obviously more overactive than the other, for this procedure furnishes a graded response—that is, the greater the defect, the greater the effect of tenotomy.

Overaction of Superior Oblique Muscles.
When this is associated with ET, a weakening procedure of one or both SO's is indicated. The procedure of choice is tenectomy. Again the effect is proportional to the degree of overaction before operation.

Comment.
In either of the above procedures, the tenotomy or tenectomy alone will affect the ET little; and, in the case of an "A" or "V" pattern, it may make the ET more constant on upward or downward gaze. Thus, one should plan to correct the ET as well as the IO or SO defect.

Overaction or Underaction of Vertical Rectus Muscles.
At times these conditions may account for unusual vertical anomalies associated with convergent strabismus. In these rarer conditions each muscle must be studied carefully—in relationship to versions and ductions—and treated accordingly, whether with recession or resection. Usually the elected procedure is done in association with a horizontal rectus operation for ET. Follow the same rules for the amount of operation as suggested for operations on the oblique muscles. Refer to the section on "Hypertropias" (page 169) for further discussion.

Divergent Strabismus

The treatment of exotropia (XT) is presented in the flowchart on pages 166–67. First, one must examine the patient to determine whether the XT is greater when the patient fixates on distant or near objects. One must always rule out pseudodivergence excess before treatment. It may become apparent whether the XT is the same at near and distant fixation with one of the following methods of examination: (1) place +3.00 diopters in front of each eye to eliminate any accommodative component and repeat the cover test, (2) occlude the drifting eye for 24 hours (Marlow's occlusion test), and (3) perform the cover test slowly. If one has determined that the XT is greater when the patient fixates on distant objects than on near objects, the patient has a divergence excess which requires surgical treatment only if there is 20 pd or more of deviation.

If there is greater than 20 pd of XT, one should determine whether the patient has an "A" or "V" pattern. If there is no "A" or "V" pattern, both LR's should be recessed 7.5 mm if the patient is more than 14 years old and 6.5 mm if the patient is less than 14 years old. If there is an "A" pattern with XT at least 15 pd greater on looking down than in the primary position and if the XT is greater than 20 pd in the primary position, then move both LR's inferiorly one muscle width and recess each to the equator (6.5 or 7.5 mm). If the XT is less than 20 pd in the primary position, move both LR's inferiorly one muscle width and recess each 1 mm. If the SO's are overactive, then do a tenectomy of both SO's and recess both LR's to the equator (6.5 or 7.5 mm). If the LR's have been previously operated on, then move each inferior rectus muscle (IR) nasally one muscle width without attempting to reoperate on the LR's to improve convergence on downgaze. If there is a "V" pattern with XT at least 15 pd greater on looking up than in the primary position and if the XT is greater than 20 pd in the primary position, then move both LR's superiorly one muscle width and recess each to the equator (6.5 or 7.5 mm). If the XT is less than 20 pd in the primary position, move both LR's superiorly one muscle width and recess each 1 mm. If the IO's are overactive, then do bilateral IO weakening procedures and recess both LR's to the equator (6.5 or 7.5 mm). If the LR's have been previously operated on, then move each

161

SR nasally one muscle width without attempting to reoperate on the LR's to improve convergence on upgaze.

If the XT is the same at near and far fixation, then recess the LR of the frankly exotropic eye to the equator (6.5 or 7.5 mm) and resect the MR 4 mm for 20 pd of deviation, 6 mm for 30 pd of deviation, and 10 mm for 50 pd of deviation. For greater than 50 pd of deviation, recess the LR to the equator (6.5 or 7.5 mm) and resect the MR 10 mm. In addition to this, if the XT is slightly greater at far fixation, recess the opposite LR to the equator (6.5 or 7.5 mm); if the XT is slightly greater at near fixation, NPC is very remote, and adduction is very poor in both eyes, resect the opposite MR 6 mm for 50 pd, 8 mm for 70 pd, and 10 mm for 90 pd (maximum).

If the XT is greater at near fixation than at distant fixation, the patient has a convergence insufficiency which is rare, and a neurologic evaluation should be considered. No surgical treatment is of lasting value. Both MR's should be resected 4 mm for 20 pd of deviation, 6 mm for 30 pd of deviation, and 8 mm for 40 pd of deviation. For 50 pd or more of deviation, recess one LR to the equator and apply the rules for correction of monocular XT.

Divergence Excess (Greater Exodeviation Far Than Near)

If far exodeviation constitutes a frank tropia or if it is intermittently greater than 20 pd, operation may be advisable. NPC must be good (better than 10 cm), and near phoria must be no more than half as great as far phoria. If far exophoria is less than 20 pd *do not* operate.

Recession of Both Lateral Rectus Muscles. The procedure of choice is bilateral LR recession to the equator; that is, 6.5 mm for 14 years old or younger and 7.5 mm for older patients.

(Refer to the chart, "Four Relatively Uncommon Strabismus Disorders," on pages 164–65.)

Monocular Exotropia

Consider that this exists if there are frank XT far and near and NPC remote (more than 10 cm), whether XT is the same far and near, a bit less near, or greater near.

Recession of Lateral Rectus and Resection of Ipsilateral Medial Rectus Muscle. The procedure of choice is recession of the LR of the exotropic eye to the equator, as defined above, plus resection of the MR on the same side as follows: resect a minimum of 4 mm for 20 pd deviation and 1 mm more for each 5 pd increase in XT to a maximum of 10 mm.

Examples:

1. For XT of 20 pd, recess LR to equator and resect MR 4 mm.
2. For 30 pd, recess LR to equator and resect MR 6 mm.
3. For 50 pd, recess LR to equator and resect MR 10 mm.
4. For more than 50 pd, recess LR to equator and resect MR 10 mm. Also, in this instance, recess the opposite LR to equator *if XT is greater at far; or* resect the opposite MR according to rule *if XT is greater at near, NPC is very remote, and adduction is very poor in both eyes.*

Convergence Insufficiency (Greater Exodeviation Near Than Far With Remote NPC)

No surgical treatment is of lasting value.

Resection of Medial Rectus Muscles. Resect both MR's 4 mm for 20 pd of XT and increase amount of resection of each muscle 1 mm/5 pd increase in XT.
Examples:

1. For a deviation of 20 pd, resect each MR 4 mm.
2. For 30 pd, resect each MR 6 mm.
3. For 40 pd, resect each MR 8 mm.
4. For 50 pd or greater, apply rule for monocular XT.

(Refer to the chart, "Four Relatively Uncommon Strabismus Disorders," on pages 164–65.)

"A" Pattern Exotropia

Operation is indicated in these cases if XT on looking down is at least 15 pd greater than in primary position; for example, 10 pd XT up, 30 pd straight ahead, and 50 pd down.

With "Normal" Oblique Action. Move both LR's down the width of one muscle and recess each to the equator *if XT is 20 pd or greater in the primary position.* Move LR's down one muscle width only but recess 1 mm to allow for loss of tissue in suturing *if XT is less than 20 pd in the primary position.*

With Definite Overaction of Superior Oblique Muscles on Versions. In this situation, if XT is 20 pd or greater in the primary position, do an intrasheath tenectomy of both SO's and recess the LR's to the equator.

FOUR RELATIVELY UNCOMMON STRABISMUS DISORDERS

	Exotropia (XT)	Orthophoria	Esotropia (ET)
	Divergence Excess (XT Greater at Far Fixation)		Divergence Insufficiency (ET Greater at Far Fixation)

Greater at Far Fixation	NPC is usually good
	Patients tolerate this well; it is the parents who note the XT
	Have good fusion at near and suppression in the distance
	Natural course:
	  1/3 get constant XT
	  1/3 stay the same
	  1/3 have spontaneous improvement
	Test: Must do Marlow's occlusion test to rule out pseudodivergence
	Age: Preschool
	Treatment: Surgery only if greater than 20 pd
	Note: When this becomes XT at near with remote NPC, treat as XT
			Usual complaint is an intermittent diplopia at far fixation
			Age: Affects older patients
			Treatment: This disorder responds quite well to prism (do not place prism over the lower part of the bifocal, at least initially).
			Resection of the LR's is not warranted unless the ET is larger (greater than 20 pd)

164

	Same at Far and Near Fixation	Greater at Near Fixation
	Convergence Insufficiency (X or XT Greater at Near Fixation)	Convergence Excess (ET Greater at Near Fixation)
	Most rare of the four disorders mentioned here. This is usually an acquired disorder related to neurologic dysfunction. Age: Affects older patients. These patients are usually quite unhappy and difficult to please. Treatment: A trial of base in prisms and, according to some, orthoptics is indicated. If this is not effective, must contemplate surgery	Most common of the four disorders mentioned here. May have a small amount of hyperopia only; may have a high AC/A ratio. Test: Must have cycloplegic refraction with test of full correction. If full correction not effective, try bifocal. If deviation persists, surgery is indicated. Age: 1½–2 years

TREATMENT OF EXOTROPIA

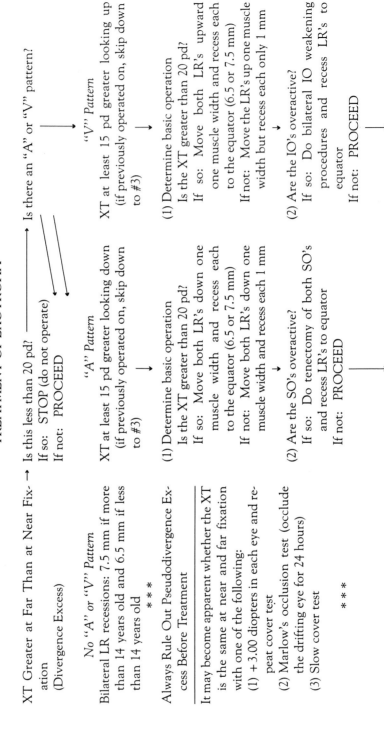

XT Greater at Far Than at Near Fixation
(Divergence Excess) →

Is this less than 20 pd?
If so: STOP (do not operate)
If not: PROCEED

No "A" or "V" Pattern
Bilateral LR recessions: 7.5 mm if more than 14 years old and 6.5 mm if less than 14 years old

* * *

Always Rule Out Pseudodivergence Excess Before Treatment

It may become apparent whether the XT is the same at near and far fixation with one of the following:
(1) +3.00 diopters in each eye and repeat cover test
(2) Marlow's occlusion test (occlude the drifting eye for 24 hours)
(3) Slow cover test

* * *

Is there an "A" or "V" pattern?

"A" Pattern
XT at least 15 pd greater looking down (if previously operated on, skip down to #3)

(1) Determine basic operation
Is the XT greater than 20 pd?
If so: Move both LR's down one muscle width and recess each to the equator (6.5 or 7.5 mm)
If not: Move both LR's down one muscle width and recess each 1 mm

(2) Are the SO's overactive?
If so: Do tenectomy of both SO's and recess LR's to equator
If not: PROCEED

"V" Pattern
XT at least 15 pd greater looking up (if previously operated on, skip down to #3)

(1) Determine basic operation
Is the XT greater than 20 pd?
If so: Move both LR's upward one muscle width and recess each to the equator (6.5 or 7.5 mm)
If not: Move the LR's up one muscle width but recess each only 1 mm

(2) Are the IO's overactive?
If so: Do bilateral IO weakening procedures and recess LR's to equator
If not: PROCEED

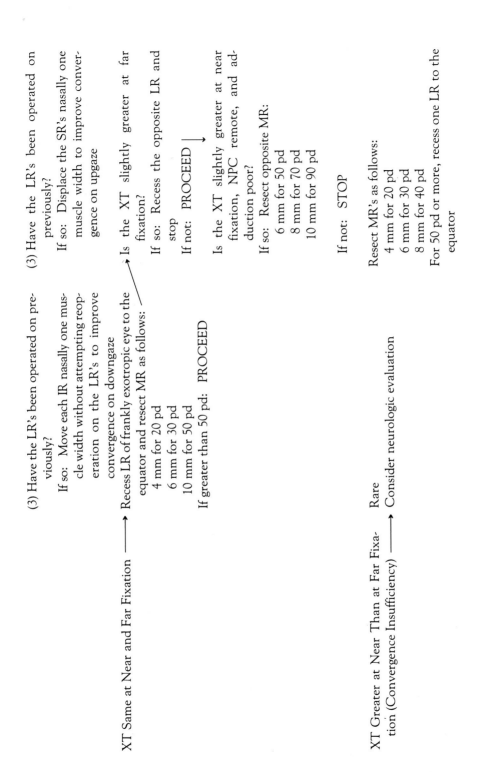

XT Same at Near and Far Fixation ──→ Recess LR of frankly exotropic eye to the equator and resect MR as follows:
4 mm for 20 pd
6 mm for 30 pd
10 mm for 50 pd
If greater than 50 pd: PROCEED

(3) Have the LR's been operated on previously?
   If so: Move each IR nasally one muscle width without attempting reoperation on the LR's to improve convergence on downgaze

──→ Is the XT slightly greater at far fixation?
   If so: Recess the opposite LR and stop
   If not: PROCEED ┐

(3) Have the LR's been operated on previously?
   If so: Displace the SR's nasally one muscle width to improve convergence on upgaze

Is the XT slightly greater at near fixation, NPC remote, and adduction poor?
   If so: Resect opposite MR:
      6 mm for 50 pd
      8 mm for 70 pd
      10 mm for 90 pd

   If not: STOP

XT Greater at Near Than at Far Fixation (Convergence Insufficiency) ──→ Rare
   Consider neurologic evaluation

Resect MR's as follows:
4 mm for 20 pd
6 mm for 30 pd
8 mm for 40 pd
For 50 pd or more, recess one LR to the equator

167

With Persistent "A" Pattern after Operation on Lateral Rectus Muscles (with Normal Oblique Action).

Move each IR nasally the width of one muscle to improve ability to converge on downward gaze.

"V" Pattern Exotropia

Operation is indicated if XT on looking up is at least 15 pd greater than in primary position; for example, 0 deviation down, 20 pd XT straight ahead, and 40 pd XT up.

With "Normal" Oblique Action.

Move both LR's upward the width of one muscle and recess to the equator *if XT in the primary position is 20 pd or greater. If XT is less than 20 pd in the primary position,* move LR's upward but recess only 1 mm to allow for loss of tissue in suturing and releasing muscles.

With Definite Inferior Oblique Overaction Bilaterally.

Recess LR's to equator for XT of 20 pd or more in primary position, and do bilateral tenotomy of IO's. If XT is less than 20 pd in primary position, do IO tenotomies only.

With Persistent "V" Pattern after Operation on Lateral Rectus Muscles (with Normal Oblique Action).

Displace SR's nasally the width of one muscle to improve ability to converge eyes.

Hypertropias

Inferior Oblique Overaction

The operation selected depends on whether the overaction is unilateral or bilateral and on the coexistence of ET or XT.

Unilateral Overaction. Tenotomy at the scleral insertion corrects as much as 20 pd of hypertropia in the field of primary action. More than 20 pd of hypertropia may require a tuck of antagonist SO also.

Bilateral Overaction. Tenotomy of both IO's is necessary. Do *both* muscles even if one is grade 1 and the other is grade 4 overactive; for, if only the greater is operated on, the lesser will show more apparent overaction after operation.

Overaction in Conjunction with ET or XT. Tenotomy of one or both IO's is indicated. This can be combined safely with operations for horizontal deviation. In our experience, IO weakening procedures performed in conjunction with LR surgery result in an adhesive syndrome in about one third of cases.

Inferior Oblique Weakness

This occurs in two principal forms.

Isolated Paresis. This lesion seldom occurs. When it does, an IO tuck of 6 to 8 mm or an advancement of the IO upward under the LR should be done.

Brown's Superior Oblique Sheath Syndrome (Apparent Paralysis of Inferior Oblique Muscle on Affected Side). The SO is the major point of attack for this disorder.
Removal or Stripping of Sheath. The SO sheath may be removed or stripped between the SR, nasally, and the point of exit of the SO from Tenon's capsule (Fig. 16).

Intrasheath Tenotomy. This operation or tenectomy is the preferred surgical procedure. Much of the sheath is destroyed during the procedure, and the eye can be rotated upward and inward by the forced duction test postoperatively.

Comment. Neither procedure is completely satisfactory, and a tuck of the ipsilateral IO may be required to enhance the result. As a rule, operate only to relieve a head turn or tilt or to enhance binocular vision, especially in the lower fields of gaze. There is a tendency for this condition to disappear as the patient becomes older.

Surgery in this condition may result in an ipsilateral IO overaction at a later date.

Superior Oblique Overaction

Unilateral Overaction. Do an intrasheath tenotomy or tenectomy (Fig. 16).

Bilateral Overaction. Do bilateral intrasheath tenotomies or tenectomies, even though one SO may be more overactive than the other.

Superior Oblique Weakness

Tuck the involved muscle temporal to SR at least 6 to 8 mm for effective result (Fig. 18). If paralysis is present, a tenotomy of the ipsilateral IO (antagonist) may be required to obtain an adequate result.

The Harada-Ito procedure may improve the intorsional function of a paretic SO.

Defects Affecting Both the Superior and Inferior Rectus Muscles

There may be IR weakness with SR overaction or IR overaction with SR weakness.

Inferior Rectus Weakness and Superior Rectus Overaction. Recess the SR to a maximum of 5 mm and resect the IR to a maximum of 5 mm.

170

Examples:

1. For hypertropia of 10 pd, recess the SR 4.5 mm and resect the IR 3.0 mm. (Recession only may suffice for lesser amounts of deviation.)
2. For hypertropia of 20 pd, recess the SR 5 mm and resect the IR 5 mm.
3. For hypertropia of more than 20 pd, recess and resect as for 20 pd; however, operation on the contralateral obliques (yoke muscles)—that is, tenotomy of the SO or tuck of the IO—may be required to obtain the desired effects.

Superior Rectus Weakness and Inferior Rectus Overaction.

The same type of treatment is indicated; that is, recess the ipsilateral IR and resect the SR maximally. (In effect, this is a *hypotropia*.)

Examples:

1. For a deviation of 10 pd, recess IR 4.5 mm and resect SR 3 mm.
2. For 20 pd, recess IR 5 mm and resect SR 5 mm.
3. For more than 20 pd, recess and resect as for 20 pd and operate on yoke muscles; that is, do a tenotomy on the contralateral IO or a tuck on the SO.

Dissociated Vertical Deviations.

Dissociated vertical divergence is most frequently seen in patients with congenital ET. It can be easily confused with other disorders of the vertical muscles. Dissociated hyperdeviation is recognized by the upward deviation of the covered (nonfixating) eye. It is almost always bilateral, so that either eye moves upward when covered and the uncovered eye moves downward to fixate. This seesaw vertical effect is observed on cross cover testing. There may also be a cyclodeviation in addition to the hyperdeviation in which the covered eye extorts and the uncovered eye intorts.

Patients with dissociated vertical deviations are asymptomatic because they do not have binocular vision. Indications for surgery are cosmetic disfigurement and deviations greater than 10 pd. No surgical approach is completely satisfactory. The recommended surgical procedures are a maximal recession of the SR (7 to 8 mm) or placement of fixation sutures 14 mm posterior to the insertion of the SR (Fäden operation). Both procedures weaken the SR. It is preferable to do the surgery bilaterally, although the quantity of surgery on each eye may be based on the amount of deviation.

TREATMENT OF VERTICAL DEVIATIONS

IO Overaction (often bilateral)	Weaken one or both IO's with tenotomy or disinsertion as needed	Do not weaken in conjunction with LR resection
IO Weakness	Is there a head turn or tilt or diplopia, especially in the lower fields of gaze? If so: PROCEED. If not: WAIT →	IO tuck of 6–8 mm or advance IO upward under the lateral rectus muscle
SO Overaction	Is there a Brown's SO sheath syndrome? If not: WAIT. If so: PROCEED	Intrasheath tenotomy or tenectomy of the SO tendon
	Weaken one or both SO's with intrasheath tenotomy or tenectomy	
SO Weakness	SO tuck of 6 to 8 mm temporal to the SR muscle or the Harada-Ito procedure	
IR Weakness and SR Overaction	Is this greater than nine to twelve months old? If not: WAIT	Recess SR 5 mm and resect IR 5 mm
SR Weakness and IR Overaction	Is this greater than nine to twelve months old? If not: WAIT	Recess IR 5 mm. If SR is −3 to −4 weak, then resect SR 5 mm
Dissociated Vertical Divergence	Is the vertical divergence less than 10 pd? If so: STOP. Do not operate. If not: PROCEED	Recess SR maximally (7–8 mm). Fäden operation may be required
Double Depressor Weakness	Move horizontal recti down to IR insertion	
Double Elevator Weakness	Move horizontal recti up to SR insertion	

Unusual Conditions

VI N Paresis or Paralysis

Under most circumstances it is wise to wait nine to twelve months after injury before proceeding with surgery in order to permit any spontaneous recovery of function. Numerous techniques have been proffered.

Lateral Rectus Resection and Medial Rectus Recession.
Recess the direct antagonist (MR) maximally (7 mm) and resect the paretic LR the amount appropriate to the degree of ET (6 to 8 mm) (previously described). The proponents of this procedure think operation should be performed as soon as an increase in ET occurs, indicating secondary contracture of the MR antagonist. This may require surgical intervention as early as 3 or 4 months postparesis. Certainly this procedure is preferred for paresis; we even prefer it for total paralysis.

Hummelsheim Operation.
Recess the MR antagonist maximally (7 mm), resect the paralytic LR maximally (10 mm), and transpose the temporal one third to one half of the SR and IR to a point just behind the LR insertion (Fig. 19).

Variations in this procedure also have been used—for instance, transposing of the *medial* one third to one half of the SR and IR temporally to assist in better abduction.

Comment. This procedure will straighten the eye, permitting elevation, depression, and adduction but little or no abduction. The eye will hold its straight position, and the patient acquires binocular vision, learning to turn the head slightly or to ignore the confusion of diplopia in the field of the paralytic LR.

Medial Rectus Recession and Transposition of the Superior and Inferior Rectus Muscles.
Recess the antagonist MR maximally (7 mm) and transpose the entire SR and IR nearly 90 degrees to be attached just above and below the LR insertion. The LR is not operated on (Fig. 20). Proponents think this procedure enhances the

chance of abduction without sacrificing elevation, depression, or adduction. An earlier suggestion was transposition of the SR and IR 45 degrees temporally with MR recession.

Comment. Both these procedures seem to have merit, especially the former; but they have failed in our hands to produce as effective a result as does the Hummelsheim procedure. Since the operations do not include LR resection, secondary deviation will be much more pronounced in the field of the paralytic LR.

Recession and Transposition (as Just Described) Plus Lateral Rectus Resection.
Proceed as in the last-described operation, but also resect the paralytic LR. However, if *all* rectus muscles are detached, the occurrence of segmental iris atrophy and anterior segment ischemia is almost certain. To *avoid* this do the LR resection six or more months later, after improved circulation to the iris via the long posterior ciliary arteries is established.

Jensen Procedure.
Recess the antagonist MR maximally (7 mm) and split the SR, LR, and IR muscles in half along their lengths and tie the lateral half of the SR to the superior half of the LR and tie the lateral half of the IR to the inferior half of the LR with nonabsorbable sutures (Fig. 21). A small scleral bite 15 mm posterior to the limbus and midway between the two joining muscle halves may be taken with each suture in order to prevent the suture from slipping anteriorly. The conjunctiva over the MR may be recessed. This procedure significantly lessens the chance of anterior segment ischemia and segmental iris atrophy.

Comment. This procedure is the simplest and most preferable of the muscle transposition operations.

See the Appendix for a comparison of the effectiveness of these procedures in the treatment of abducens muscle palsy.

IV N Paresis or Paralysis

Wait nine to twelve months to permit improvement; if none occurs, operation on the paretic SO, alone or in conjunction with operation on the direct antagonist, is in order. Head tilt and torsional defect usually are present. The three-step test should be used to logically evaluate any isolated cyclovertical muscle palsy. Step 1: Which eye had hypertropia in the primary position? Step 2: Which direction of gaze, right or left, increases the hypertropia? Step 3: Does the Bielschowsky head tilt test to the right or to the left increase the hypertropia? The eye with the paretic SO will

TREATMENT OF CRANIAL NERVE VI PALSY

Has the sixth nerve palsy been present for nine to twelve months? If not: STOP. If so: PROCEED ⟶ Is the palsy partial or complete?

↓

Partial or Complete
Recess the conjunctiva
Recess the MR of the involved eye 7 to 8 mm
Resect the LR as follows:
  4 mm for 20 pd ET
  6 mm for 30 pd ET
  8 mm for 40 pd ET
  10 mm for 60 pd ET

Complete
Jensen procedure:
1. Recess conjunctiva
   Recess MR 7 to 8 mm
   Divide LR, SR, and IR
2. Suture temporal SR and upper LR slips together. Attach these to the sclera about 15 mm from the limbus at 45 degrees
3. Suture temporal IR and lower LR slips together. Attach these to the sclera about 15 mm from the limbus at 45 degrees

have a hypertropia on primary position, adduction, and head tilt to the ipsilateral side. Some prefer to operate on the yoke muscle or its direct antagonist, but this seldom helps the torsion abnormality as much as does operation on the oblique muscles themselves.

Paresis Only. The choice of operation depends on the deformity.
Minimal Inferior Oblique Overaction with Minimal Superior Oblique Weakness. In this instance, do a tuck of the paretic SO tendon. A tuck of 8 mm usually suffices (Fig. 18).
Moderate or Marked Inferior Oblique Overaction. If antagonist IO is overactive, and SO paresis is not obvious, do only a tenotomy of the IO (Fig. 15).
No Vertical Component, But a Torsional Component. The Harada-Ito procedure is usually performed bilaterally for bilateral SO palsy in which there is no vertical deviation, but where there is an excyclotropia of 7° to 20° in primary position that increases in midline downgaze (Fig. 18).

Paralysis. Successive procedures are available.
Superior Oblique Tuck and Inferior Oblique Tenotomy. Do a maximal tuck of the SO (10 mm) combined with tenotomy of the IO. Usually this procedure is adequate.

175

TREATMENT OF CRANIAL NERVE IV PALSY

Has the fourth nerve palsy been present for nine to twelve months? If not: STOP. If so: PROCEED ⟶ Is the palsy due to trauma? If so: Check for bilateral involvement which is frequent

Is the palsy partial or complete?

Partial

Is the palsy low grade and is the IO overactive?
If so: Weaken IO only
If not: PROCEED

Is the palsy grade 3 with an overactive IO or weak SR?
If so: Weaken IO and tuck SO 6 to 8 mm
If not: PROCEED

Recess contralateral IR 5 to 6 mm if tuck is not desired

Harado-Ito procedure is useful if there is no vertical component, but only a torsional component causing excyclotropia

Complete

IO weakening plus maximum SO tuck (10 to 12 mm)
If not effective: PROCEED

Recess contralateral IR 5 to 6 mm if the above is not competely effective

Contralateral Inferior Rectus Recession. Recess the contralateral IR 5 to 6 mm if hyperdeviation persists after SO tuck and IO tenotomy. This is a secondary procedure.

Contralateral Superior Rectus Resection. Resect the contralateral SR if the deviation still is not corrected. This is a tertiary procedure.

Congenital III N Paralysis

This defect, usually accompanied by ptosis, is difficult to correct by surgery.

Hummelsheim Type of Procedure. Recess LR to equator (10 to 12 mm), resect paralytic MR maximally (8 to 10 mm), and transpose medial halves of SR and IR to reinsert at MR insertion (Fig. 19).

Hummelsheim Type Plus Transposition of Superior Oblique Tendon. Proceed as just described but also transpose SO tendon to insert at MR insertion (Fig. 19). Free SO tendon nasal to SR and resect it sufficiently so that it is taut when attached at point of MR insertion. This may help to splint eye in straight-ahead position. In any case, abduction is about all that is present anyway. We have found it unnecessary to fracture the trochlea for this procedure.

Recession and Resection. Recess LR to equator (10 to 12 mm) and resect MR maximally (8 to 10 mm). This usually is not sufficient and it does not help the *hypo*tropia which often exists. This may be combined with a transposition of the SO tendon to improve its effectiveness. A traction suture from the MR insertion through the skin and medial canthal ligament and tied in position for 10 days to 2 weeks may prevent scarring and return of the eye to its original position.

Comment. Treat ptosis after other muscle defects have been corrected.

Other Isolated Defects of Rectus Muscle

Muscle transposition procedures of the Hummelsheim type have been used effectively for MR absence or paralysis if isolated. For injured SR or IR, leading to paralysis or loss of muscle, a maximal recession of the direct antagonist combined with resection of the paralytic muscle and transposition of slips from the MR and LR to the insertion of the defective muscle.

TREATMENT OF CRANIAL NERVE III PALSY

Has the third nerve palsy been present for nine to twelve months? If not: STOP. If so: PROCEED ⟶ Does the palsy completely or partially involve the third nerve muscles?

Partial
Recess LR 10 to 12 mm
Recess conjunctiva
Resect MR maximally (8 to 10 mm)
↓
Eyelid surgery will be required secondarily
↓
Exposure of the globe is the chief problem after eyelid surgery

Complete
Recess LR 10 to 12 mm
Recess conjunctiva
Resect MR maximally (8 to 10 mm)
Sever SO nasal to SR and attach at MR insertion under tension
Then, reattach MR
↓
Traction suture to hold eye adducted 2 weeks may be used

177

have proved effective in at least holding the eye in a near primary position without compromising the actions of the nonparetic muscles.

Ophthalmopathy of Graves' Disease

Defects may result which try the expertise of even the most qualified muscle surgeons. Usually there is a unilateral or bilateral weakness of elevation with contracture of the IR's, often combined with weakness of abduction and contraction of the MR's. When the general status of the patient is stable, muscle surgery may be instituted.

Recession of Contracted Muscles.

Recess the contracted muscles maximally (5 to 7 mm for SR or IR, 5.5 mm for MR's and 7.5 mm for LR's). In IR recession, dissect the IR away from the IO as far posteriorly as possible to prevent retraction of the lid. (Forced duction tests reveal an inability to move the globe away from the contracted muscle even with a hook under the insertion.) Placement of the sutures must be done with extreme care so that the globe is not perforated by the needle. When the muscle is freed from its insertion, it may be difficult to re-advance it adequately to give the desired degree of recession. However, a greater recession (6 mm or more) may be desirable in this condition.

Resection of Antagonistic Muscles.

Resect the muscles which are direct antagonists to the contracted muscles maximally (4 mm for vertical rectus muscles and 8 to 10 mm for horizontal rectus muscles).

Comment.

Do not operate on more than three rectus muscles of one eye. Use procedures on the oblique muscles to aid elevation or depression if rectus surgery seems insufficient.

Usually it is best to base operation on muscles obviously affected and to reoperate in six months if proper alignment is not obtained. In this unusual condition the eyes may obtain a better position slowly after the initial operation. We have found the following general rules useful: When an IR is contracted, recess it alone; if an MR is contracted, recess it only; if an SR is contracted, recess it *and* resect the direct antagonist.

If results of the initial operation are obviously inadequate, one may reoperate the same muscles very soon (within a day or two) to obtain better binocular alignment. Usually it is best to add to the resection rather than to the recession, since the latter was maximal at the first operation. If more than two or three days elapse, it is best to wait four to six weeks before reoperating.

TREATMENT OF GRAVES' OPHTHALMOPATHY

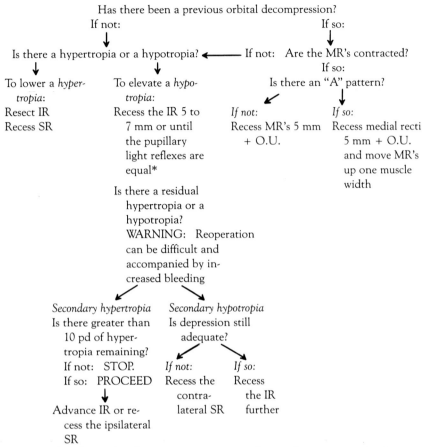

Has there been a previous orbital decompression?

If not: If so:

Is there a hypertropia or a hypotropia? ◄——— If not: Are the MR's contracted?

                                                                              If so:

To lower a *hyper-*   To elevate a *hypo-*   Is there an "A" pattern?
tropia: tropia:
Resect IR   Recess the IR 5 to   *If not:*   *If so:*
Recess SR   7 mm or until   Recess MR's 5 mm   Recess medial recti
                              the pupillary   + O.U.   5 mm + O.U.
                              light reflexes are   and move MR's
                              equal*   up one muscle
                                                                     width
                           Is there a residual
                              hypertropia or a
                              hypotropia?
                              WARNING: Reoperation
                              can be difficult and
                              accompanied by in-
                              creased bleeding

Secondary hypertropia   *Secondary hypotropia*
Is there greater than   Is depression still
   10 pd of hyper-   adequate?
   tropia remaining?
If not: STOP.   *If not:*   *If so:*
If so: PROCEED   Recess the   Recess
                           contra-   the IR
Advance IR or re-   lateral SR   further
cess the ipsilateral
SR

Graves' ophthalmopathy *always* causes restriction of a muscle—not a paresis of an
   antagonist.
Vigorously strip away the aponeurosis to the lower eyelid prior to recession of the IR
   to prevent and alleviate eyelid retraction.
Consider referral in these patients: these patients notoriously yield unpredictable results, and surgery may be complicated by excessive bleeding.
The most affected muscle is the IR, then the MR, then the SR. The LR is seldom
   affected.
The order of procedures in Graves' ophthalmopathy is (1) decompression, (2) muscles,
   (3) lid.

---

*With the use of general and local anesthesia, alignment of the pupillary light reflexes can
be helpful in achieving good alignment in Graves' disease, unlike most horizontal deviations.

As suggested for other procedures, allow six months or more to pass before operating on the fourth rectus muscle. See the Appendix for further details.

Retraction Syndromes

Duane's Syndrome. If binocular vision is present in the straight-ahead position and to the uninvolved side, do no surgery. If a head turn is necessary to acquire and maintain binocularity, a recession of the MR maximally will help to place the binocular field so that head turn is less noticeable or unnecessary. Do not expect to prevent retraction of the globe on adduction or to aid abduction. If the eye is divergent, reverse the process.

Strabismus Fixus. A fixed squint is an unusual problem, but an attempt can be made to weaken the contracted muscles and strengthen opposing rectus muscles in an effort to produce relatively straight eyes. Since the globe itself is rather rigid, even with the rectus muscles loosened, the chance of success is reduced considerably. Great difficulty may be encountered in reattaching the muscles, especially on recession.

PART FIVE

Complications and Technical Errors

Complications

Many complications, minor and major, can occur during or after operations on ocular muscles. Some general principles of treatment are outlined in this chapter, but the best preventatives are careful surgical technique and knowledge of anatomy.

Suture Reaction

This occurs to a mild degree in nearly all instances in which absorbable material is used and even more frequently after reoperations if such material was used during the initial procedure. In our experience the reactions are milder when coated Vicryl suture material is used than they are with other absorbable materials; also, chromic suture causes less reaction than does plain suture. The onset may occur about ten days to three weeks postoperatively, and the reaction usually presents as a yellow-red lump over the suture site. Reaction subsides rather promptly, but healing may be aided by the use of topical steroids and hot compresses. Rarely, a persistent piece of suture needs to be excised before complete healing occurs. It is best to alert the parents to this possible eventuality. Suture reactions are almost nonexistent with the suture material currently used.

Tenon's Capsule Cyst

A cyst may form when a knuckle of capsular material is caught between conjunctival sutures. The contained fluid may be clear or milky. Often cysts subside spontaneously in a few days or weeks, but some require excision with closure of the conjunctiva over the wound. Decompressing the cyst by puncture may be tried first.

Persistent Redness and Edema

The site of the incision may remain red and edematous because of improper closure of the conjunctiva or, more often (in the case of young patients), because of closure of Tenon's capsule instead of conjunctiva or suturing of Tenon's capsule to conjunctiva. The result is a dull appearance of the healed surface. Further surgery to close the conjunctiva properly is in order.

Muscle Adhesions and Scarring

These result from undue trauma at operation, bleeding that persists after closure, or undue suture reaction. Formation of adhesions to the sclera, to Tenon's capsule, or to other muscles may result in immediate or delayed secondary ocular deviations (undercorrections or overcorrections), limitation of motion in various fields of gaze, and even enophthalmos. Repeated operations may lead to loss of the conjunctiva and Tenon's capsule; thus, new adhesions may alter the position of the globe simply because the covering tissues cannot relax.

Reoperation to free adhesions is necessary when limitation of motion is found; otherwise, a greater defect (muscular or cosmetic) results. Leaving bare sclera from the limbus to the muscle insertion may be required to relax the conjunctiva sufficiently to permit the globe to assume a normal position. The use of Gelfilm or other substances to reduce scarring has proved mostly ineffective in our experience.

Extreme care is necessary in freeing muscles or adhesions from the sclera or Tenon's capsule since the globe may be perforated if a hook is pushed too vigorously in an attempt to isolate a muscle, or a muscle may be severed unknowingly. Proper orientation is to be maintained always to avoid isolating the wrong muscle. Sharp dissection may help to isolate cleavage planes more readily than does stripping the adhesions, and bleeding should be controlled as one progresses. Excessive use of cautery will result in even more scarring. Identify carefully each structure as it is isolated and orient the globe before reattaching muscles. Measure from the limbus for desired amounts of recession or reattachment of a resected muscle when reoperating. *Prevention* of adhesions by careful and gentle handling of tissue at the first operation is the best practice.

Anterior Segment Ischemia and Iris Atrophy

Anterior segment ischemia and segmental iris atrophy may result from severing all four rectus muscles completely. At least one muscle or portions of two muscles must remain intact to maintain an adequate blood supply to the iris and anterior segment. Even for children one should allow time (four to six months) for establishment of adequate collateral circulation before detaching the remaining rectus muscle or slips of muscle.

Loss of Vision

This rare but unfortunate complication can result from excess bleeding into the muscle cone with resultant undue pressure on the posterior globe. This has occurred in only two of our patients, in each of whom there appeared to be a posterior uveitis, which cleared to leave a pigmented scar in the macular area with reduced central acuity. Undue trauma to the posterior portion of the globe during muscle surgery could conceivably cause a similar circumstance. The treatment is prevention by exercise of good surgical techniques.

Perforation of the Globe

Most frequently this occurs at the time of reattachment of a muscle to the sclera. Today's ophthalmic needles are so sharp that one must use gentle pressure only when slipping the needle into the sclera. The needles should be positioned tangential to the sclera at all times and never perpendicular to the scleral surface when suturing. The needle must be "seen" just beneath the surface as it is passed for 3 mm or so for an adequate "hold." Placement of sutures in the muscle prior to detaching it from the sclera requires diligence since the sclera can be perforated easily. If the sclera is perforated completely so that vitreous extrudes, the pupil should be well dilated and the retina thoroughly examined by indirect ophthalmoscopy, and any damage should be repaired immediately. Fortunately the site of injury is usually in the periphery so that vision is not compromised. Infection is rare if sterile precautions are maintained; however, one may feel more at ease if large doses of antibiotics are used prophylactically for a few days.

A large perforation made with muscle hook, scissors, or knife may occur. This is most likely when one is operating on muscles scarred down or thickened from previous operations. Closure and repair of such larger wounds should be immediate, and the operation should be discontinued except for repair of the defect. Antibiotics may be of even more importance than for smaller perforations. For either a minor or major perforation, placement of a rectus muscle over the wound adds an extra baffle to support the repair.

After three or four weeks one may again attack the muscles to accomplish the original goal. We have yet to observe a retinal detachment or a fulminating infection of the globe resulting from a simple perforation with a surgical needle when the above precautions were followed.

Technical Errors

Surgery of Wrong Muscle

Careful orientation of each muscle operated on must be made before suturing or releasing it. Since the eye may roll upward under anesthesia, it is somewhat more difficult to orient the horizontal rectus muscle planes. The globe should be rotated downward by traction with forceps at the lower limbus, or upper as for placement of a superior rectus suture for cataract surgery, and the traction suture then can be placed properly. Some surgeons think traction sutures at both the 12 o'clock and 6 o'clock positions maintain better orientation than does a single suture at the limbal area adjacent to the muscle to be operated on.

After isolation of the muscle, traction with the muscle hook also ensures proper identification. If one is still in doubt, isolate adjoining rectus muscles and measure the distance of insertion from the limbus, which is quite consistent unless prior surgery has been performed.

Improper Line of Reattachment

When placing sutures, for a recession in particular, the proper line of attachment can be lost. Marking the sclera with a dye such as methylene blue at points above and below the muscle before detaching it from the sclera will help to prevent this error. Since the globe can rotate easily when one grasps the upper or lower edge of the original site of insertion, have the assistant hold one edge while the surgeon holds the other to prevent false localization. If one is to transposition a muscle for "A" or "V" patterns, this precaution is very important. Reattach the muscle parallel to the limbus; in doing this one should remember the usual line of attachment of the vertical rectus muscles and attempt to duplicate this in reattachment.

Twisting of the muscle on itself will compromise the desired result. If a double-armed suture is used, leave one arm shorter to identify the upper or lower muscle border. In any case, draw the muscle forward before reattaching it to be certain that it is in a proper relationship.

186

Overcorrection

Whether the cause of overcorrection is too much surgery, a "lost" muscle, or scarring after operation, an additional operation usually is in order. This applies for horizontal and vertical muscles.

Too Much Surgery. It has been our experience that one can judge the result of an operation quite accurately the next day if a recession-resection procedure was performed. The eye may converge a bit more later, or elevate or depress better, but usually an overcorrection from too much surgery will remain. If the operation consisted of bilateral recessions or a single recession, time may prove beneficial. In any event, one should allow several weeks to pass to assess the final outcome before reoperating. Usually too much recession or too generous a resection has been done. If there is evident weakness in the field of action of the recessed muscle, readvancement to the original site of insertion may suffice. Frequently, however, one must anticipate more than this, and a very satisfactory solution is a marginal myotomy of the resected muscle (see operative procedures illustrated in Figure 14) plus readvancement of the recessed muscle. For deviations greater than about 20 pd, maximal recession of the resected muscle (see prior text) with advancement of the recessed muscle may be necessary. Some surgeons prefer to attack the contralateral unoperated yoke muscles, but we think the situation should be treated on the basis of "how it looks," or as an original procedure, and that one should correct a weakness or overaction as it exists. Naturally one may need to operate on the yoke muscles if the defect is uncorrected by reoperation or if numerous prior procedures have distorted anatomy or position to such an extent that one has no alternative.

If an IO or SO tuck is too effective, release of the tuck partially or fully must be done.

The same procedures usually apply to overcorrection resulting months or years after a successful operation.

"Lost" Muscle. This is a rare occurrence if the operation was properly performed in the first place. However, the defect usually is evident immediately (by the next day or within a few hours). There is an inability to rotate the globe in the field of action of the involved muscle— in this instance, the recessed muscle. One should reoperate immediately to identify and reattach the muscle since healing of the tissues is amazingly rapid. If one elects to wait, a period of three to four weeks should elapse to permit time for tissue swelling to subside.

Free the tissues gently, stop bleeding as it occurs, and usually the muscle can be identified easily lying against Tenon's capsule in a somewhat retracted position. Reattachment at the originally intended site is satisfactory if operation is repeated in a day or two. If reoperation is delayed, a greater deviation may have ensued, requiring advancement of the muscle to its original insertion or even weakening of the resected muscle.

Postoperative Scarring. This important problem, already discussed under "Complications," is reconsidered here because it frequently manifests as overcorrection and because it does relate to technique. It may result from poor hemostasis, bleeding after closure, improper dissection, suture reaction, improper closure, or individual patient peculiarity. The position of the eye may be satisfactory for weeks before gradual evidence of overcorrection appears. Forced duction tests will often give a clue to the position of the defect.

Treatment is difficult. Release of scar tissue and adhesions around the muscle, above to Tenon's capsule or below to the sclera, may free the globe adequately. Prevention of future scarring may present a problem, however. The use of Gelfilm between muscle and sclera or muscle and Tenon's capsule may help, but it is difficult to keep it in position. Silastic material or a Supramid sleeve may be inserted in these positions and secured with fine sutures; the material is inert and creates little reaction.

If simple releasing of adhesions does not free the globe adequately, recession of the resected muscle or advancement of the recessed muscle may be necessary. Remember that scarring of the IO to a resected LR or of the SO to a resected SR might result in rotary defects. In such instances free the oblique muscle from the undersurface of the rectus muscle before reattaching it to the sclera, whether for resection or recession.

Scarring as a result of suture reaction may present a similar situation. The use of inert nonabsorbable suture material, such as Dacron or nylon, will allay future reactions of this type.

Repeated procedures may compromise the result by scarring or loss of conjunctiva. Forced duction tests may show that the globe is held by shortened tissues other than muscle. When these are dissected free, the globe can be rotated readily. To prevent future problems the conjunctival edge can be attached to the sclera so that it covers just the muscle attachment, leaving several millimeters of bare sclera between it and the limbus. This is quickly covered by epithelium, which permits a smooth and effective surface. Conjunctival grafts may be required in some instances, but usually they are less satisfactory. Here, as in the case of other complications, prevention by careful attention to dissection, suturing of muscle, and wound closure is best.

Undercorrections

Probably a more frequent complication than overcorrection, under-correction results from too little surgery, from loosening of a resected muscle, or from scarring.

Insufficient Surgery. As noted before, the result from a reces-sion-resection operation usually is apparent the day after operation and alters little thereafter. If a symmetrical operation (bimedial or bilateral recessions or resections) was performed, however, a gradual improvement often can be expected. Thus, in most instances three to six months should pass before further surgery is contemplated. At reoperation the situation must be assessed as if it were a new one; that is, if a full recession of a muscle was performed at first, and this muscle seems correct in its action, operate on its yoke muscle or further resect its antagonist. If the recessed muscle seems overactive still, a marginal myotomy is useful or further recession to the maximal amount (see earlier text) combined with further resection is in order. If the previously operated eye seems to move adequately on versions, or if further operation on those muscles is unde-sirable for any reason, operate on the yoke muscle, basing the amount of operation on the rules described in "Surgical Procedures."

If a bimedial recession resulted in an undercorrection, a marginal myotomy of one MR plus a resection of the ipsilateral LR may suffice; if maximal recession of the MR was not done, it should be done at reopera-tion in addition to the LR resection. Similar procedures may be used on the opposite eye if the deviation still persists. When a bilateral LR reces-sion fails to correct an exodeviation, application of similar principles will correct the defect.

If a weakening procedure of the IO is inadequate, further surgery to detach the muscle from the sclera (tenotomy) or more recession is neces-sary. If one anticipates a greater need, strengthen the antagonist also. Fur-ther surgery to weaken an SO tendon is fraught with more problems; if a primary intrasheath tenotomy was deemed adequate, strengthening the IO antagonist or operation on the yoke muscle (opposite IR) is necessary.

Loosening of Resected Muscle. This is a rather rare occur-rence. If it is present soon after operation (within 24 to 48 hours), reat-tachment at the original insertion is in order. A "lost" resected muscle may be more difficult to find either at the time of operation or later. Usu-ally it can be found lying against Tenon's capsule if a careful and calm search is made. If the muscle cannot be found, fashion a tendon from a

189

HORIZONTAL MUSCLE REOPERATIONS

Previous ET
Is the patient overcorrected
or undercorrected?

Undercorrected
Was the previous operation unilateral or bilateral?

Overcorrected
Was the previous operation unilateral or bilateral?

Unilateral
Is the MR recessed maximally? If not: Recess further. If so: Perform Z tenotomy of the MR and resect the LR as per the previous formula. NOTE: One must go past the midline with each of two slices to make a Z tenotomy effective

Bilateral
Are the MR's recessed maximally?
If not: Recess further
If so: Resect LR's

Unilateral
If there was a prior recession-resection, advance MR and recess LR. Treat as a new problem

Bilateral
If prior bimedial procedure and adduction is weak, advance the MR's and recess one LR. If deviation is greater than 50 pd, may recess both LR's

Recess the conjunctiva over the recessed muscle only. Conjunctival recession is reserved for secondary procedures and very large deviations

Previous XT

Is the patient overcorrected or undercorrected?

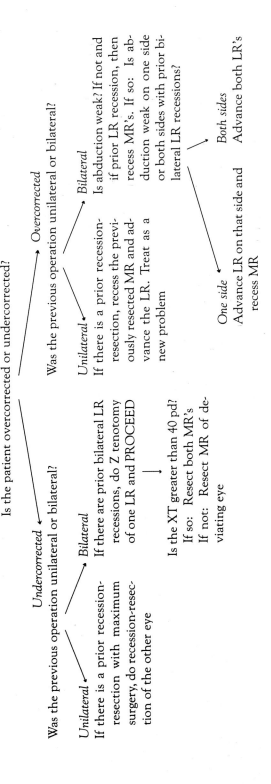

Undercorrected

Was the previous operation unilateral or bilateral?

Unilateral
If there is a prior recession-resection with maximum surgery, do recession-resection of the other eye

Bilateral
If there are prior bilateral LR recessions, do Z tenotomy of one LR and PROCEED

Is the XT greater than 40 pd?
If so: Resect both MR's
If not: Resect MR of deviating eye

Overcorrected

Was the previous operation unilateral or bilateral?

Unilateral
If there is a prior recession-resection, recess the previously resected MR and advance the LR. Treat as a new problem

Bilateral
Is abduction weak? If not and if prior LR recession, then recess MR's. If so: Is abduction weak on one side or both sides with prior bilateral LR recessions?

One side
Advance LR on that side and recess MR

Both sides
Advance both LR's

191

tongue of Tenon's capsule or attach a band of Silastic to the intended point of insertion on the globe and to the orbital fascia. The resulting defect in ocular position should be minimal if the unoperated eye is the fixing eye. Also one may use a muscle transposition procedure in an effort to hold the globe in better position. One should employ a procedure of the Hummelsheim type if another rectus muscle has been operated on, or wait four months or more until better collateral circulation to the iris is established if full muscle transpositions are preferred. Either procedure may be applied for any "lost" rectus muscle.

If late weakening of the muscle is apparent, reoperation to check the area of attachment is necessary. Readvance the muscle to its intended insertion if it is not located there; if this is deemed inadequate to correct the existing muscle imbalance, further resection may be required.

Postoperative Scarring.   The same principles apply as outlined for overcorrection.

Comments

Ordinarily, with undercorrection or overcorrection, the *resulting deviation must be approached as a new situation*, and the muscles to be operated on are chosen on the basis of the principles discussed in previous sections.

PART SIX

Anesthesia for Strabismus Surgery

by
Allan B. Gould, Jr., M.D.
Consultant, Department of Anesthesiology,
Mayo Clinic and Mayo Foundation

Anesthesia for Strabismus Surgery

The anesthetic management of patients having strabismus surgery presents some unique problems that involve not only the anesthesiologist but also the surgeon. An example of this is the oculocardiac reflex, a common challenge in the management of these patients. It is most promptly and most successfully treated by identification of the problem by the anesthesiologist and removal of the stimulus by the surgeon. Other frequently encountered problems that are related to the anesthetic are those associated with outpatient surgery, special considerations for pediatric patients, and anesthetic complications such as postoperative nausea and vomiting, laryngeal edema, and malignant hyperpyrexia. Although these problems are not unique to strabismus surgery, they must be considered when determining the anesthetic. Although this procedure can be done with the patient under local anesthesia, this discussion will be centered on the use of general anesthesia for pediatric patients because more anesthetic problems are encountered in this group of patients.

Anesthetic Concerns in Pediatric Patients

Because fluid requirements are usually calculated on the basis of the patient's weight, the smaller the patient, the more critical is the determination of fluid needs. Adequate hydration during and after the surgical procedure warrants careful attention. Fluid administration during the procedure is based on 4 ml/kg per hour starting at the time of the last oral feeding for children weighing 10 kg or less. For each kilogram of body weight from 10 to 20, an additional 2 ml/kg per hour is added, and for each kilogram above 20, 1 ml/kg per hour is given. One half of the calculated requirement is given in the first hour, and the balance is given throughout the procedure.

Preoperatively, children up to 6 months of age may have clear fluids until four hours before administration of the anesthetic. Patients up to 5 years of age should take nothing by mouth after midnight except clear fluids, which they may have up to six hours before administration of the anesthetic. Children over 5 years of age should have nothing by mouth after midnight.

195

Premedication to prepare the pediatric patient for anesthesia must be determined on an individual basis. These drugs are given to decrease secretions and to sedate the patient. Reassurance by the parent and informing the child about the pending surgical experience by the physician are usually more helpful than drugs in obtaining a young patient's cooperation. The needle used for premedication may initiate fear and apprehension, so many anesthesiologists avoid premedication unless it is specifically indicated. If one anticipates that secretions will be a problem, atropine (0.1 mg/10 kg up to 0.6 mg) may be warranted; however, doses usually used in premedication will not be adequate to reliably block the vagal portion of the oculocardiac reflex. If sedative drugs seem to be warranted, 1 mg/kg of meperidine is usually adequate. Ketamine given intramuscularly or rectally administered thiopental or methohexital are very useful either for quieting a child who is unable or unwilling to cooperate or for induction agents.

Because the airway is not readily accessible to the anesthesiologist during strabismus surgery, endotracheal intubation is necessary to ensure a secure airway for the patient during the procedure. Because the walls of an endotracheal tube must be thick enough to resist kinking, the internal diameter of small tubes is disproportionately smaller than the external diameter. The external diameter of the tube must allow it to fit easily through the larynx; however, the internal diameter must be as large as possible to minimize the resistance to gas flow and to make it more difficult to become plugged with mucus. An excessively large endotracheal tube predisposes the patient to laryngeal edema.

Monitoring the pediatric patient during anesthesia for strabismus surgery typically includes use of a blood pressure cuff, a precordial or esophageal stethoscope, a cardioscope, a thermometer with axillary probe, and an oxygen monitor. Because of the relatively large surface area of children, maintenance of body temperature during anesthesia is very important and warrants a warm operating room. During strabismus surgery, when the body is well covered with drapes and the procedures are not prolonged, hypothermia is not as great a problem as it is during procedures in which large body surfaces are exposed for prolonged periods.

Anesthetic Techniques in Pediatric Patients

Three commonly used pediatric anesthetic techniques for strabismus surgery are (1) ketamine induction followed by a muscle relaxant, intubation, and maintenance with an inhalation agent; (2) barbiturate induction, muscle relaxant, intubation, and maintenance with an inhalation agent; and (3) inhalation induction with a volatile agent, intubation without a muscle relaxant, and maintenance with the same inhalation agents.

196

The technique that uses ketamine has the advantage that the drug can be administered by intramuscular injection. This procedure avoids the need for both an inhalation induction and a venipuncture in the awake patient. Intravenous barbiturate induction is both a pleasant and quick way to start the anesthetic once the venipuncture is completed. An inhalation induction can be rapid and enables one to avoid using succinylcholine for intubation. My personal preference is for an inhalation induction of anesthesia in children. Halothane has been the inhalation agent of choice because it is pleasant to breathe in the concentrations necessary to induce anesthesia.

The Oculocardiac Reflex

Oculocardiac reflex is often associated with strabismus surgery. It is initiated by traction on the extraocular muscles, most commonly the medial rectus, or by pressure on the globe. It may cause quite sudden and severe cardiovascular changes that warrant immediate treatment. This reflex is made up of afferent trigeminal parasympathetic fibers going to the cardioinhibitory centers of the brain and efferent vagal fibers that cause bradycardia and depress sinoatrial node rhythmicity. This reflex may manifest as bradycardia, atrioventricular block, bigeminal rhythm, or hypotension.

As indicated earlier, the first line of treatment is communication between the surgeon and anesthesiologist and removal of the stimulus. Fortunately, this reflex usually fatigues rapidly and may require no further treatment. Occasionally a reflex will persist throughout the procedure.

If the reflex persists and drug therapy becomes necessary, mephentermine will usually resolve the problem quickly and permanently. It stimulates cardiac output by increasing the myocardial contractile force without producing ventricular arrhythmias. Vagal blockade with atropine is a logical method of treatment; however, the effect is often of short duration and repeated doses are sometimes necessary.

When the oculocardiac reflex continues to be a problem,[3] a retrobulbar block may be necessary.

Anesthetic Complications

Children should not have had an upper respiratory infection within the 2 weeks preceding surgery in order to minimize laryngospasm after removal of the endotracheal tube. This spasm is caused by thick pulmonary secretions that are coughed up as the patient awakens. Strabismus surgery is an elective procedure, and the patient should be in the best possible health to provide for an uneventful and uncomplicated use of a general anesthetic.

Laryngeal edema is most frequently of concern in children up to 5 years of age. One millimeter of edema at the cricoid level in these small children may result in an obstruction of up to 75 per cent of the airway. This complication usually becomes evident within the first two hours after removal of the endotracheal tube and must be treated promptly. It is seen more frequently in females and after prolonged intubation. A croupy cough, inspiratory stridor, intercostal retraction, tachypnea, or tachycardia may serve as the initial warning. Intravenous administration of dexamethasone (2 to 3 mg), intermittent positive-pressure administration of racemic epinephrine, and good humidification are all useful[4] in the treatment of postintubation laryngeal edema.

It has been suggested that patients having strabismus surgery have a higher incidence of malignant hyperpyrexia. This complication is infrequent; however, succinylcholine and the halogenated inhalation agents have been demonstrated to trigger it. Successful treatment depends both on early recognition and on prompt, vigorous treatment. An unexplained tachycardia is the most common early warning of the onset of malignant hyperpyrexia. Rigidity after the administration of succinylcholine is also a frequent first sign. One must not wait for temperature elevation to make the diagnosis and to initiate therapy. Early administration of dantrolene, a hydantoin derivative that is specific in the management of this problem, can greatly increase the patient's chance for survival. In general, treatment consists of vigorous cooling, cessation of the administration of volatile anesthetic agents, and appropriate supportive measures and laboratory studies. Delay in the diagnosis of malignant hyperpyrexia may result in death. Sixty to 70 per cent of patients with malignant hyperpyrexia died before the introduction of dantrolene. If the diagnosis is delayed and the patient survives, sequelae such as disseminated intravascular coagulopathy, acute tubular necrosis, hypothermia, muscle necrosis, or anoxic neurologic damage may occur.

The incidence of nausea and vomiting is high in patients undergoing surgery for strabismus. This is of special concern when the patient is an outpatient, and it may ultimately lead to hospitalization. Droperidol in doses of 75 μg/kg is reported[1] to be safe and effective in decreasing the incidence and severity of postanesthetic vomiting.

General Anesthesia for Outpatients

Current economic pressures are resulting in an increase in the number of strabismus procedures being done on an outpatient basis. Although this practice provides a considerable saving to the patient in the total cost for the procedure, it also provides problems such as (1) inappropriate oral intake before anesthesia, (2) added precautions necessary for an early diagnosis of laryngeal edema, and (3) residual drug effects in the dismissed patient.

A major reason for admitting children to the hospital on the day before surgery has been to ensure that oral intake is appropriately limited before the administration of the anesthetic. The child who has surgery on an outpatient basis occasionally succeeds in circumventing the usual measures that allow him to have an empty stomach when anesthesia is induced. Careful instructions to the parents explaining why fasting is important can eliminate this problem and allow no greater risk of vomiting and aspiration for the outpatient than for the inpatient.

The primary reason for postoperative hospitalization of a child who has received endotracheal anesthesia is to allow for the early diagnosis of laryngeal edema.

Another major concern regarding general anesthesia for outpatients is that of residual drug effect. Although the most obvious effects of the inhalation agents will have dissipated soon after the patient arrives in the recovery room, judgment and coordination will be compromised for a prolonged period. Adults should be specifically prohibited from driving a motor vehicle until the next day. Epstein[2] reported that 30 per cent of licensed drivers who are dismissed as outpatients after general anesthesia drive within 12 hours of the administration of an anesthetic. Drugs such as diazepam, droperidol, and promethazine have a long action and should not be routinely used to premedicate outpatients.

References

1. Abramowitz, M. D., Oh, T. H., Epstein, B. S., Ruttimann, U. E., and Friendly, D. S.: The antiemetic effect of droperidol following outpatient strabismus surgery in children. Anesthesiology 59:579–583, 1983.
2. Epstein, B. S.: Recovery from anesthesia (editorial). Anesthesiology 43:285–289, 1975.
3. Jedeikin, R. J., and Hoffman, S.: The oculocardiac reflex in eye-surgery anesthesia. Anesth. Analg. 56:333–334, 1977.
4. Koka, B. V., Jeon, I. S., Andre, J. M., MacKay, I., and Smith, R. M.: Postintubation croup in children. Anesth. Analg. 56:501–505, 1977.

Appendix

New Extraocular Muscle Clamp*

John A. Dyer, M.D.

A small vascular clamp with the serrated edges at a 45° angle holds extraocular muscles firmly without crushing. The instrument may be applied from either side of the muscle.

The instrument is manufactured by V. Mueller and Company, 6600 W. Touhy Ave., Chicago, IL 60648.

Summary

A small vascular clamp with the serrated edges at a 45° angle holds extraocular muscles firmly without crushing.

---

*Dyer, J. A.: New extraocular muscle clamp. Published with permission from The American Journal of Ophthalmology. 79:330, 1975. Copyright by the Ophthalmic Publishing Company.

Appendix

Inferior Oblique Surgery: Experience at the Mayo Clinic From 1960 to 1981*

Thomas W. Jones, Jr, M.D.; David A. Lee, M.D.; John A. Dyer, M.D.

Three hundred thirty-seven patients underwent inferior oblique dis-insertions at the Mayo Clinic Rochester, Minn, from 1960 to 1981. Versions and hyperdeviations in the primary position were recorded preoperatively and postoperatively. The criteria of a successful result were (1) correction of diplopia, (2) correction of hyperdeviation in the field of action of the inferior oblique, and (3) correction of versions in adduction. Clinical failure was reflected in persistence of hyperdeviation in primary gaze and persistence of overaction of the inferior oblique muscle in adduction. A successful result was found in 88% of primary inferior oblique disinsertions. For secondary inferior oblique overaction, a successful result was found in 72% of patients. We have found that inferior oblique disinsertion is a safe, fast, reliable, and effective weakening procedure with good results. (*Arch Ophthalmol* 1984; 102:714-716)

Since the time of Duane's[1] description of weakening the inferior oblique muscle by a myotomy at the origin to Parks' graded recession,[2] there has been continued controversy regarding the procedure of choice for weakening the inferior oblique muscle. The proponents of recession[2-7] regard this as the procedure of choice primarily because of (1) the ability to achieve a graded response, (2) a longer-lasting response, (3) the lack of residual weakness, and (4) the avoidance of the adhesive syndrome. Those who advocate myectomy[8-11] promote it for its simplicity and effectiveness. Proponents of disinsertion stress similar advantages without the disadvantages of a longer operating time and the increased risk of complications.[12-15]

*Jones, T. W., Jr., Lee, D. A., and Dyer, J. A.: Inferior oblique surgery: experience at the Mayo Clinic from 1960 to 1981. Arch Ophthalmol 102: 714-16, 1984. (By permission.)

204

This retrospective study was undertaken to review the results of inferior oblique disinsertions performed between 1960 and 1981 at the Mayo Clinic, Rochester, Minn. We attempted to quantitate the effect of inferior oblique disinsertion with preoperative and postoperative versions and hyperdeviation in the primary gaze.

Method

Clinical data were collected on 337 patients ranging in age from 7 months to 76 years. Some patients were followed up for as long as 19 years, and some were seen only once, at two weeks after surgery. All patients who were seen up to two weeks postoperatively were included in the study. All operations were performed by the same surgeon (J.A.D.), and all preoperative and postoperative versions and hyperdeviations were measured by the same orthoptic technician.

The indications for weakening the inferior oblique muscle included (1) isolated unilateral or bilateral primary inferior oblique overaction and (2) secondary unilateral or bilateral inferior oblique overaction.

Patients were grouped as having either primary or secondary inferior oblique overaction. They were further classified as having unilateral and bilateral involvement, and statistical analysis was done by considering these four groups of patients.

Statistical analysis used the $2 \times 2\chi^2$ and Fisher's exact tests for comparing discrete variables (ie, sex, family history of strabismus, presence of associated factors, presence of symptoms, history of surgery, reoperations for overcorrection and undercorrection, and presence of asymmetry). The two-sample t test and Wilcoxon's rank sum test were used for comparing continuous variables (ie, age at the time of surgery, duration of overaction, preoperative and postoperative hypertropia in primary gaze, preoperative and postoperative versions, and duration of follow-up). Comparisons were made between unilateral or bilateral involvement and primary and secondary overaction, with preoperative and postoperative (using paired tests) values. Spearman's r test was used to determine whether any significant correlations existed between preoperative and postoperative values for hypertropia in primary gaze and versions. A level of $P < .05$ was considered to be statistically significant.

Results

Of the 295 patients with primary inferior oblique muscle overaction, 131 had unilateral overaction and 164 had bilateral overaction (Table 1). Approximately half of the patients were male and half were female in both groups. A family history of strabismus was noted in a significantly larger number of patients in the bilateral overaction group (17%) than in the unilateral overaction group (2%). However, diplopia, head turn or tilt, or chin up or down occurred more frequently in the unilateral over-action group (21%) than in the bilateral overaction group (5%). No significant differences were found between the two groups in regard to associated factors (ie, trauma, Graves' disease, and prematurity), history of extraocular muscle surgery, and reoperations for overcorrection or undercorrection. Undercorrections were more common in both groups as an indication for reoperation.

The primary unilateral overaction group was significantly older at the time of surgery (mean age, 20 years) than the primary bilateral overaction group (mean age, 6 years). Also, the duration of inferior oblique muscle overaction was longer in the unilateral group (mean, six years) than in the bilateral group (mean, four years). Preoperative hypertropia in primary gaze was greater in the unilateral group (mean, 9 PD) than in the bilateral group (mean, 2 PD). However, no difference was found between the two groups in the amount of postoperative hypertropia. There was a significant decrease in the amount of hypertropia in the unilateral group, from a preoperative mean of 9 PD to a postoperative mean of 2 PD. This change was not seen in the bilateral group. Versions were significantly changed in both groups, from preoperative mean values of 1.5 PD in the unilateral group and 1.6 PD in the bilateral group to postoperative mean values of -0.2 PD in the unilateral group and 0 PD in the bilateral group. The postoperative values for versions were significantly different between the unilateral and bilateral groups. The follow-up duration was the same in both groups (mean, four to five years).

Of the 42 patients with secondary inferior oblique muscle overaction, 36 had unilateral overaction and six had bilateral overaction (Table 2). The frequency of a family history of strabismus was greater in the unilateral group than in the bilateral group. No differences between the two groups were found in sex, associated factors, symptoms, prior surgery, or reoperations. As for the primary overaction group, the secondary overaction group had undercorrection as the more common cause of reoperation in both unilateral and bilateral groups.

The age at the time of surgery, duration of overaction, amount of hypertropia in primary gaze preoperatively and postoperatively, versions preoperatively and postoperatively, and duration of follow-up were comparable in the unilateral and bilateral groups. Both groups had significant differences between preoperative and postoperative values for the amount of hypertropia and versions. In the unilateral group, hypertropia

206

Table 1. Primary Inferior Oblique Muscle Overaction*

	Unilateral (n = 131)	Bilateral (n = 164 [328 Eyes])
Sex		
M	72 (55)	88 (54)
F	59 (45)	76 (46)
Family history†	3 (2)‡	28 (17)
Associated factors	10 (8)‡	19 (12)‡
Symptoms†	27 (21)‡	9 (5)‡
Prior surgery	27 (21)‡	37 (23)‡
Reoperations		
Overcorrection	1 (1)	0
Undercorrection	13 (10)	19 (12%)
Total	14 (11)‡	19 (12)‡
Age, yr†	20.1 ± 20.4‡	6.0 ± 6.2‡
Duration of overaction, yr†	6.2 ± 8.5	4.0 ± 3.6
Hypertropia in primary gaze, PD		
Preoperative†	8.6 ± 8.1‡§	2.0 ± 4.0‡
Postoperative	1.6 ± 2.7‡§	2.0 ± 3.8
Versions, PD		
Preoperative	1.5 ± 0.6§	1.6 ± 0.7§
Postoperative†	−0.2 ± 0.6§	0.0 ± 0.5†§
Follow-up, yr	4.0 ± 4.4	4.9 ± 4.5

*Some data (lower half of table) are shown as mean ± SD. Other values are number (percent) of patients.

†Statistically significant (P < .05) difference between unilateral and bilateral involvement.

‡Statistically significant (P < .05) difference between primary and secondary involvement (within unilateral or bilateral group).

§Statistically significant (P < .05) difference between preoperative and postoperative values.

Appendix

Table 2. Secondary Inferior Oblique Muscle Overaction*

	Unilateral (n = 36)	Bilateral (n = 6 [12 Eyes])
Sex		
M	19 (53)	4 (67)
F	17 (47)	2 (33)
Family history†	17 (47)‡	0
Associated factors	15 (42)‡	4 (67)‡
Symptoms	20 (56)‡	2 (33)‡
Prior surgery	3 (8)‡	1 (17)
Reoperations		
Overcorrection	1 (3)	0
Undercorrection	8 (22)	3 (50)
Total	9 (25)‡	3 (50)‡
Age, yr	31.3 ± 18.9‡	29.5 ± 22.6‡
Duration of overaction, yr	6.3 ± 5.9	6.3 ± 5.3
Hypertropia in primary gaze, PD		
Preoperative	17.6 ± 12.7‡§	11.5 ± 10.0‡§
Postoperative	3.5 ± 4.7‡§	2.0 ± 2.5§
Versions, PD		
Preoperative	1.4 ± 0.7§	1.7 ± 0.8§
Postoperative	−0.3 ± 1.0§	−1.2 ± 1.0‡§
Follow-up, yr	2.8 ± 3.5	1.4 ± 1.9

*Some data (lower half of table) are shown as mean ± SD. Other values are number (percent) of patients. Statistical interpretation of the data from the secondary bilateral inferior oblique muscle overaction group should be made cautiously because of the small sample size (six patients).

†Statistically significant (P < .05) difference between unilateral and bilateral involvement.

‡Statistically significant (P < .05) difference between primary and secondary involvement (within unilateral or bilateral group).

§Statistically significant (P < .05) difference between preoperative and postoperative values.

208

decreased from a preoperative mean of 18 PD to a postoperative mean of 4 PD. A similar decrease was seen in the bilateral group: 12 PD preoperatively to 2 PD postoperatively. The amount of overaction seen in versions also decreased from 1.4 to −0.3 PD for the unilateral group and from 1.7 to −1.2 PD for the bilateral group. Significant positive correlations were found between preoperative and postoperative hypertropia and versions for primary unilateral and bilateral inferior oblique muscle overactions and secondary unilateral inferior oblique muscle overaction.

Significant differences were found between unilateral primary and secondary overactions in family history of strabismus, associated factors, symptoms, prior surgery, reoperations, age at the time of surgery, and preoperative and postoperative hypertropia in primary gaze (Tables 1 and 2). Bilateral primary and secondary overaction groups were significantly different in associated factors, symptoms, reoperations, age at the time of surgery, preoperative hypertropia in primary gaze, and postoperative versions (Tables 1 and 2).

Table 3 shows the frequency of preoperative and postoperative asymmetries of bilateral inferior oblique muscle overaction. Preoperatively, asymmetric hypertropia in primary gaze was significantly less in primary than in secondary overaction. Asymmetric versions in primary overaction were significantly less postoperatively (18%) than preoperatively (28%). Statistical conclusions are difficult to make for the secondary bilateral overaction group because of the small sample size.

Table 3. Asymmetry of Bilateral Inferior Oblique Muscle Overaction*

	No. (%) of Patients	
	Primary (n = 164)	Secondary (n = 6)
Hypertropia in primary gaze		
Preoperative†	45 (27)	6 (100)
Postoperative	51 (31)	3 (50)
Versions		
Preoperative	46 (28)‡	3 (50)
Postoperative	29 (18)‡	2 (33)

*Statistical interpretation of the data from the secondary bilateral inferior oblique muscle overaction group should be made cautiously because of the small sample size (six patients).

†Statistically significant ($P < .05$) difference between primary and secondary involvement.

‡Statistically significant ($P < .05$) difference between preoperative and postoperative values.

Complications

The most frequent complication in this study was persistent overaction; it was seen in 10% of the primary overactive inferior oblique group and 26% of the secondary overactive inferior oblique group. Hypotropia was seen in less than 1% in both the primary and secondary overactive groups. The entity described in 1972 by Parks[2] as the "adhesive syndrome" was believed to be a specific syndrome related to disinsertions and myectomies of the inferior oblique muscle. There were no instances of an isolated disinsertion with the complication described by Parks. One instance of persistent hyperdeviation was found to be related to adhesions surrounding the superior rectus. In this case, the patient had a fourth cranial nerve palsy with a corresponding inferior oblique overaction. In addition to a disinsertion, a tuck of the superior oblique, myotomy of the superior rectus, and a muscle transposition of the medial and lateral rectus muscles were also performed.

In the two cases of hypotropia, adhesions were believed to be a factor but, again, multiple muscles were subjected to surgery.[16] It seems more plausible to assume that postoperative restrictions result from (1) too little or too much dissection of Tenon's capsule and (2) improper muscle manipulation.[17] Inherent in any extraocular muscle surgery is the potential risk of adhesions. One should always strive for good surgical technique, with meticulous dissection.

A phenomenon often seen with unilateral weakening procedures is the occurrence of inferior oblique overaction in the contralateral eye. An interesting explanation for this phenomenon was offered by Fleming.[18] He stated that when the inferior oblique is surgically weakened, the unopposed ipsilateral superior oblique muscle causes intorsion, which is compensated for by the contralateral inferior oblique. The increased stimulation of the contralateral inferior oblique muscle causes it to become overactive. Indeed, in 12% of the primary unilateral inferior oblique disinsertions in this study a contralateral inferior oblique overaction developed and required surgical treatment. The average time from the first disinsertion to the contralateral second disinsertion was approximately 23 months.

Comment

In this retrospective study of 337 patients from 1960 to 1981, approximately 87% of all patients had an acceptable result. Parks[2] in 1972 reported comparable results with recession. Recently, Edwards and Hess[11] also reported excellent results with myectomy. With the inherent problems associated with reproducing precise statistics regarding the deviation in the cardinal fields of gaze, we believed, from a practical standpoint, that the reoperative rate, along with hyperdeviation in the primary gaze and versions, provided us with an important clinical criterion for success.

The results of a properly done inferior oblique weakening procedure are generally good, whether the operation is recession, myectomy, or disinsertion. A question that each physician must then ask himself is "What are the rewards and risks of any given surgical procedure?" Both myectomy and recession are inherently longer and more involved than disinsertion, although all are equivalently successful. Acceptance of one approach over another often takes more than reasoning; it takes time. In our hands, disinsertion has withstood the test of time.

References

1. Duane A: Tenotomy of inferior oblique and consideration of the conditions that may call for the operation, abstracted. *Br Med J* 1906;2:1867–1868.
2. Parks MM: The weakening surgical procedures for eliminating overaction of the inferior oblique muscle. *Am J Ophthalmol* 1972;73:107–122.
3. White JW: Surgery of the inferior oblique at or near the insertion. *Trans Am Ophthalmol Soc* 1942;40:118–121.
4. Dunnington JH, in discussion, White JW: Recession of the inferior oblique muscle. *Arch Ophthalmol* 1943;29:1034.
5. Brown HW: Surgery of the oblique muscles, in Allen JH (ed): *Strabismus Ophthalmic Symposium.* St Louis, CV Mosby Co, 1950, pp 401–422.
6. Fink WH: Oblique muscle surgery from the anatomic viewpoint. *Am J Ophthalmol* 1951;34:261–281.
7. Dunlap EA: Inferior oblique weakening: Recession, myotomy, myectomy, or disinsertion? *Ann Ophthalmol* 1972;4:905–912.
8. Scobee RG: *The Oculorotary Muscles,* ed 2. St Louis, CV Mosby Co, 1952, pp 475–477.
9. Schlossman A: Surgery of the inferior oblique. *Eye Ear Nose Throat Monthly* 1955;34:328–329.
10. McNeer KW, Scott AB, Jampolsky A: A technique for surgically weakening the inferior oblique muscle. *Arch Ophthalmol* 1965; 73:87–88.

11. Edwards WC, Hess JB: Inferior oblique surgery. *Ann Ophthalmol* 1982;14:831–834.

12. Dyer JA: Tenotomy of the inferior oblique muscle at its scleral insertion: An easy and effective procedure. *Arch Ophthalmol* 1962;68:176–181.

13. Dyer JA, Duke DG: Inferior oblique weakening procedures. *Int Ophthalmol Clin* 1976;16(Fall):103–112.

14. Costenbader FD, Kertesz E: Relaxing procedures of the inferior oblique: A comparative study . *Am J Ophthalmol* 1964;57:276–280.

15. Cooper EL, Sandall GS: Recession versus free myotomy at the insertion of the inferior oblique muscle: Comparative analysis of the surgical correction of overaction of the inferior oblique muscle. *J Pediatr Ophthalmol* 1969;6:6–10.

16. Dyer JA: Some pitfalls with simultaneous inferior oblique tenotomy (disinsertion) and lateral rectus resection. *J Pediatr Ophthalmol* 1973;10:47–53.

17. Price RL: Role of Tenon's capsule in postoperative restrictions. *Int Ophthalmol Clin* 1976;16 (Fall):197–207.

18. Fleming AW: Overactive inferior oblique muscle. *Ann Ophthalmol* 1977;9:1515–1517.

Bilateral Medial Rectus Muscle Recession and Lateral Rectus Muscle Resection in the Treatment of Congenital Esotropia*

David A. Lee, M.D., and John A. Dyer, M.D.

In a retrospective study of 36 patients with congenital esotropia treated surgically by bilateral medial rectus muscle recession and lateral rectus muscle resection, we found that 22 patients (61%) had not required further surgery and that 14 patients (39%) had required further corrective surgery. Seven of these 14 patients had overcorrections and seven had undercorrections. Patients who required a second operation were significantly younger (mean age, 12 months) than those who did not (mean age, 23 months). The most common second surgical procedure was bilateral tenotomy or disinsertion of the inferior oblique muscle.

Bilateral medial rectus muscle recession and lateral rectus muscle resection is useful in severe (50 prism diopters or more) congenital esotropia. The surgical success rate may be improved with bilateral inferior oblique muscle disinsertions or tenotomies in patients with inferior oblique muscle overaction. Accurate preoperative examinations in patients old enough to cooperate may help avoid overcorrection and undercorrection.

Congenital esotropia begins before the age of 6 months. It is usually characterized by a large deviation that is nonaccommodative in origin. The generally accepted treatment is surgical alignment of the eyes, usually a combined recession of the medial rectus muscle and resection of the lateral rectus muscle in the nonfixating eye (asymmetrical) or a recession of both medial recti muscles (symmetrical).

Von Noorden, Isaza, and Parks,[1] Ing and associates,[2] and Foster, Paul, and Jampolsky[3] reported that satisfactory surgical realignment with the initial surgical attempt occurs in 40% to 80% of cases. Secondary sur-

*Lee, D. A., and Dyer, J. A.: Bilateral medial rectus muscle recession and lateral rectus muscle resection in the treatment of congenital esotropia. Published with permission from The American Journal of Ophthalmology. 95:528–535, 1983. Copyright by the Ophthalmic Publishing Company.

gery for overcorrection and undercorrection is common. Bietti and Bago-lini,[4] Arruga,[5] and Taylor[6] reported the incidence of undercorrection to be from 20% to 50%, and Arruga,[5] Taylor,[6] Cooper,[7] Landolt and Koenig,[8] and Windsor[9] reported that of overcorrection to be from 4% to 8%. Cooper,[7] Landolt and Koenig,[8] and Windsor[9] noted that symmetrical and asymmetrical surgery produced similar frequencies of overcorrection and undercorrection.

We conducted a study to analyze the results of bilateral medial rectus muscle recessions and lateral rectus muscle resections in the treatment of congenital esotropia.

Subjects and Methods

We conducted a retrospective review of charts for all bilateral medial rectus muscle recessions and lateral rectus muscle resections performed by one of us (J.A.D.) for congenital esotropia at the Mayo Clinic from 1968 to 1981. All 36 patients satisfied the following criteria: onset of esotropia before the age of 6 months; nonaccommodative and constant esotropia; crossed fixation pattern; limited abduction to both sides; no previous eye surgery; and absence of organic visual and central nervous system disorders. Other patients with congenital esotropia of less than 50 prism diopters and full rotation underwent other surgical procedures.

The following variables were measured and analyzed: age at initial surgery; sex; family history of strabismus; birth history; amount of deviation before and after surgery (by Hirschberg estimate, Krimsky test, or cover test with prisms); refractive error (by cycloplegic retinoscopy); amount of medial rectus muscle recession and lateral rectus muscle resection; binocular fusion (by a Worth four-dot test); stereopsis (by Titmus test); duration of follow-up; and secondary surgery for overcorrection and undercorrection. Visual acuity was difficult to determine in such young patients. All the patients were able to hold fixation with either eye at the time of surgery and apparently had equal vision. If amblyopia was present or suspected, the fixating eye was patched before surgery until either eye was able to hold fixation.

The surgical approach consisted of a 4.5- to 5-mm recession of the medial rectus muscle and a 4- to 8-mm resection of the lateral rectus muscle of each eye. In some instances of overaction of the inferior oblique muscles, determined preoperatively, bilateral disinsertions or tenotomies of the inferior oblique muscles were performed in addition to the horizontal muscle surgery. The goal of the initial surgical procedure was full mechanical alignment in the primary position.

The collected data were analyzed statistically. We used the 2×2 chi-square test and Fisher's exact test to compare sex, birth history, family history, and tenotomy or disinsertion of both inferior oblique muscles in patients who had significant deviations after surgery and who required second operations (Group 1) with those patients who did not require second operations (Group 2). We used the two-sample t-test and the Wilcoxon rank sum test to compare age, degree of preoperative esotropia, refractive error, duration of follow-up, amount of medial rectus recession and lateral rectus resection, and the absolute postoperative deviation of reoperation and no reoperation. Also, we used the two-sample t-test and the rank sum test to compare age, degree of preoperative esotropia, amount of postoperative deviation, and refractive error in patients who had final peripheral fusion and in those who had no peripheral fusion, as measured by the Worth four-dot test. Spearman's r test was used to determine whether any significant correlations existed between the following variables: age and preoperative deviation, age and postoperative deviation, refractive error and preoperative deviation, refractive error and postoperative deviation, preoperative deviation and postoperative deviation, duration of follow-up and postoperative deviation, amount of medial rectus muscle recession and preoperative deviation, amount of medial rectus muscle recession and postoperative deviation, amount of lateral rectus muscle resection and preoperative deviation, and amount of lateral rectus muscle resection and postoperative deviation. We considered a $P < .05$ level to be statistically significant.

Results

Of the 36 patients who underwent bilateral medial rectus muscle recessions and lateral rectus muscle resections (Table 1), 14 (39%) required and underwent further surgery at a later date. The mean age ($\pm$ S.E.) of the patients in Group 1 was 12.4 ± 1.9 months, whereas that of the patients in Group 2 was 23.4 ± 3.7 months. The difference was statistically significant. As expected, the absolute postoperative deviation in Group 2 was much smaller, 3.8 ± 1 degrees, than that in Group 1, 12.6 ± 1 degrees. This difference was also statistically significant. Borderline statistical significance was found in birth history, with Group 1 including three abnormal births and Group 2 including none. We found no significant differences between the two groups in regard to sex, family history of strabismus, amount of preoperative esotropia, refractive error, amount of medial rectus muscle recession, amount of lateral rectus muscle resection, tenotomy or disinsertion of both inferior oblique muscles, or duration of follow-up.

Appendix

Table 1 Summary of Clinical Data

Clinical Data	No. or Mean ± S.E.	
	Group 1	Group 2
Patients	14 (39%)	22 (61%)
Sex		
Male	8	8
Female	6	14
Birth history*		
Normal and full-term	11	21
Normal and full-term with		
cesarean section	0	1
Breech delivery	1	0
Premature	2	0
Family history of strabismus		
Contributory	3	7
Noncontributory	11	15
Age (mos)†	12.4 ± 1.9	23.4 ± 3.7
Presurgical deviation (degrees)	27.5 ± 3.0	31.1 ± 1.8
Refractive error (diopters)	+2.04 ± 0.22	+2.43 ± 0.24
Amount of recession of medial rectus		
muscle (mm)	4.68 ± 0.07	4.63 ± 0.05
Amount of resection of lateral rectus		
muscle (mm)	5.64 ± 0.29	5.95 ± 0.28
Tenotomy or disinsertion of both		
inferior oblique muscles	2	6
Absolute postsurgical deviation		
(degrees)†	12.6 ± 1.0	3.8 ± 1.0
Duration of follow-up (yrs)	3.12 ± 0.48	4.35 ± 0.67

*Borderline significance by Fisher's exact test (one-tailed), P = .05.
†Statistically significant by unpaired t-test and unpaired Wilcoxon test, P < .05.

Table 2 shows the secondary surgical procedures that the patients in Group 1 underwent. Seven patients (50%) had overcorrections and significant residual exotropia, and seven had undercorrections and significant residual esotropia. Five of seven patients with overcorrections and about three of seven with undercorrections underwent bilateral inferior oblique disinsertions or tenotomies. Almost one half (six of 14) of the patients in Group 1 (17% of all the patients in this study) underwent a third surgical procedure.

Table 3 shows the fusional data. None of the 36 patients in this study had central fusion (determined by a positive result of the Titmus

Table 2 Summary of Secondary Procedures

Secondary Procedures	No. of Patients	
Total	14	(39%)
Second procedure for overcorrection	7	(19.4%)
Disinsertion or tenotomy of both inferior oblique muscles	5	
Recession of both lateral recti muscles	2	
Recession of one lateral rectus muscle	1	
Marginal myotomy of one lateral rectus muscle	1	
Second procedure for undercorrection	7	(19.4%)
Disinsertion or tenotomy of both inferior oblique muscles	3	
Disinsertion or tenotomy of one inferior oblique muscle	1	
Resection of both lateral recti muscles	1	
Resection of one lateral rectus muscle	3	
Marginal myotomy of both medial recti muscles	2	
Marginal myotomy of one medial rectus muscle	3	
Third surgical procedure required	6	(17%)

stereoscopic visual acuity test recorded in the chart). Only 15 of 22 charts for the patients in Group 2 contained Worth four-dot test results. Six of the 15 patients (40%) had peripheral fusion on the basis of results of this test, and nine (60%) had no peripheral fusion. The difference in the amount of postoperative deviation between patients who had fusion and those who did not have fusion was statistically significant. We found no significant differences in regard to age, refractive error, or amount of pre-operative deviation between those with and those without fusion. Only two of 14 patients (14%) in Group 1 had peripheral fusion by the Worth

Table 3 Peripheral Fusion in Patients in Group 2

	No. or Mean ± S.E.	
Clinical Data	Fusion	No Fusion
Patients*	6 (40%)	9 (60%)
Age (mos)	26.0 ± 8.0	23.6 ± 5.7
Refractive error (diopters)	+2.04 ± 0.36	+2.39 ± 0.36
Preoperative deviation (degrees)	27.5 ± 2.8	35.6 ± 2.9
Postoperative deviation (degrees)†	0.7 ± 0.7	6.7 ± 2.0

  *The results of a Worth four-dot test were available for only 15 of the 22 patients who did not require further surgery.

  †Statistically significant difference ($P < .01$).

four-dot test after the second surgical procedure. None of the patients who underwent a third surgical procedure had peripheral fusion.

A statistically significant ($P < .02$) positive correlation (Spearman's $r = .448$) was found between preoperative and postoperative deviation. We found borderline statistically significant ($P \approx .05$) correlations between the amount of preoperative deviation and medial rectus muscle recessions, amount of lateral rectus muscle resection and postoperative deviation, and age and postoperative deviation. No significant correlations were found between age and preoperative deviation, refractive error and preoperative deviation, refractive error and postoperative deviation, amount of medial rectus muscle recession and postoperative deviation, amount of preoperative deviation and lateral rectus muscle resection, or postoperative deviation and duration of follow-up.

Discussion

Congenital strabismus is a common disorder. Taylor[6] estimated the incidence to be at least 50% in the overall strabismus population. According to Costenbader,[10] congenital esotropia is usually defined as constant esotropia with onset between birth and 6 months of age, and the group is heterogeneous, including different causes and prognoses. Therefore, results of treatment for this condition are difficult to evaluate critically. Bair[11] expressed the belief that a deviation of 10 prism diopters or less is necessary for the development of single binocular vision during infancy or early childhood. It is generally accepted that surgery is necessary to straighten congenitally esotropic eyes. Both the time that surgery should be performed and the best surgical procedure have aroused controversy.

There are basically two different schools of thought on the best time to operate. One school, represented by Ing and associates,[2] Taylor,[6,12,13] Costenbader,[14] Parks,[15] and Ing,[16] believes that surgery should be done within the first two years of life and preferably during the first year of life. This reasoning goes back to Chavasse,[17] who believed that early single binocular vision is important in the development of normal binocular reflexes. Other reasons for operating early are that surgical risk has been reduced by improved anesthetic procedures, that long-standing strabismus causes secondary changes in the extraocular muscles, conjunctiva, and Tenon's capsule, making later surgical correction more difficult, and that psychologic effects must be considered.

Another school of thought, represented by von Noorden, Isaza, and Parks,[1] Foster, Paul, and Jampolsky,[3] Arruga,[5] and Fisher, Flom, and Jampolsky,[18] is that surgery should be performed when the child is 2 years of age or older. This is based on Worth's[19] assumption that a congenital defect of fusion faculty is the cause of squint. Totally normal binocular vision has never been documented in a congenitally esotropic patient, regardless of the age at which surgical correction was performed. Also, because it is difficult to examine an infant accurately, the incidences of undercorrection and overcorrection may be increased and associated vertical anomalies may be overlooked. In a comparison of results of operations performed before and after the patients were 18 months old, von Noorden, Isaza, and Parks[1] found no differences in deviation and binocular function.

In our study, patients who underwent further surgery had an average age of 12 months, whereas those who did not have further surgery had a mean age of 23 months. This difference was statistically significant. Patients who had peripheral fusion, determined by the Worth four-dot test, were slightly older than those who had no fusion. However, this difference was not significant. There was a borderline significant correlation between age and postoperative deviation. Patients who were older at the time of initial surgery tended to have smaller residual deviations. This result suggested that bilateral recession of the medial rectus muscle and resection of the lateral rectus muscle are more effective in older patients with congenital esotropia. This finding may have been the result of more accurate preoperative testing in older patients (2 years of age) that led to better surgical correction. Sex, birth history, family history of strabismus, presurgical deviation, and refractive error were not significant predictors of surgical success. As expected, patients in whom peripheral fusion developed had significantly smaller postoperative deviations than those in whom it did not develop.

The most common surgical procedures used to treat congenital esotropia are a combined recession of the medial rectus muscle and resection of the lateral rectus muscle in one eye (asymmetrical) and a recession of both medial recti muscles (symmetrical). Each procedure has its disadvantages in the correction of a large-angle esotropia. In severe esotropia, an asymmetrical procedure can cause nonconcomitance and a symmetrical procedure can cause convergence impairment. As Cooper[7] and Windsor[9] noted, there is little difference between the results of symmetrical and asymmetrical surgery. Bietti and Bagolini,[4] Arruga,[5] Taylor,[6] Cooper,[7] Landolt and Koenig,[8] and Windsor[9] reported that procedures tend to result in more undercorrections than overcorrections. In this series of bilateral medial rectus muscle recession and lateral rectus muscle resection, the success rate was 61% (22 of 36), which was comparable to rates reported by von Noorden, Isaza, and Parks,[1] Ing and associates,[2] and Foster, Paul, and Jampolsky,[3] who used other surgical procedures.

Appendix

One half of the patients in Group 1 had overcorrections and one half had undercorrections. Overcorrections were more likely to occur in patients with less preoperative esotropia, and undercorrections were more likely to occur in patients with more preoperative esotropia. Although statistically significant, this correlation did not allow us to predict the postoperative outcome clinically, because of the large degree of variability. Bilateral medial rectus muscle recession and lateral rectus muscle resection avoids nonconcomitance and lessens the possibility of convergence impairment and should, therefore, be considered in the early treatment of severe (50 prism diopters or more) congenital esotropia. Operating on four horizontal muscles enhances the chance for fusion and results in fewer undercorrections. However, four-muscle procedures in patients with less than 50 prism diopters of deviation may result in a greater number of overcorrections.

According to Ing and associates,[2] Foster, Paul, and Jampolsky,[3] Windsor,[9] and Parks,[15] overaction of one or both inferior oblique muscles and dissociative double hyperdeviations are common in patients with congenital esotropia. This was also the case in our study. Eight of 36 patients (22%) underwent bilateral tenotomy or disinsertion of the inferior oblique muscles at the time of initial surgery. Six of the eight did not require further surgery. Of the 14 patients who underwent a second surgical procedure, nine had inferior oblique tenotomies or disinsertions. Procedures weakening the inferior oblique muscles should probably be done more often during the initial surgical procedure when there is evidence of inferior oblique overaction.

In view of our findings, we recommend bilateral recession-resection procedures when the amount of deviation is 25 degrees (50 diopters) or more. A useful guide is to recess both medial recti muscles 5 mm from the original insertion and resect both lateral recti muscles 5 mm for 50 prism diopters; resect both lateral recti muscles 6 mm for 60 prism diopters and an additional 1 mm for each 10 prism diopters of esotropia to a maximum of 8 mm. If one or both inferior oblique muscles are overactive, they should be weakened at the same time, preferably bilaterally.

References

1. von Noorden, G. K., Isaza, A., and Parks, M. E.: Surgical treatment of congenital esotropia. Trans. Am. Acad. Ophthalmol. Otolaryngol. 76:1465, 1972.
2. Ing, M., Costenbader, F. D., Parks, M. M., and Albert, D. G.: Early surgery for congenital esotropia. Am. J. Ophthalmol. 61:1419, 1966.

3. Foster, R. S., Paul, T. O., and Jampolsky, A.: Management of infantile esotropia. Am. J. Ophthalmol. 82:291, 1976.

4. Bietti, G. B., and Bagolini, B.: Problems related to surgical overcorrections in strabismus surgery. J. Pediatr. Ophthalmol. 2:11, 1965.

5. Arruga, A.: Surgical overcorrections. J. Pediatr. Ophthalmol. 2:15, 1965.

6. Taylor, D. M.: Congenital strabismus. The common sense approach. Arch. Ophthalmol. 77:478, 1967.

7. Cooper, E. L.: The surgical management of secondary exotropia. Trans. Am. Acad. Ophthalmol. Otolaryngol. 65:595, 1961.

8. Landolt, E., and Koenig, F., Jr.: Zum operativ überkorrigierten Begleitschielen. Ophthalmologica 131:266, 1956.

9. Windsor, C. E.: Surgically overcorrected esotropia. A study of its causes, sensory anomalies, fusional results, and management. Am. Orthopt. J. 16:8, 1966.

10. Costenbader, F. D.: Infantile esotropia. Clinical characteristics and diagnosis. Am. Orthopt. J. 18:5, 1968.

11. Bair, D. R.: Infantile esotropia. Sensory evaluation and results. Am. Orthopt. J. 18:15, 1968.

12. Taylor, D. M.: How early is early surgery in the management of strabismus? Arch. Ophthalmol. 70:752, 1963.

13. _____: Is congenital esotropia functionally curable? Trans. Am. Ophthalmol. Soc. 70:529, 1972.

14. Costenbader, F. D.: Infantile esotropia. Trans. Am. Ophthalmol. Soc. 59:397, 1961.

15. Parks, M. M.: Infantile esotropia. Summary and conclusions. Am. Orthopt. J. 18:19, 1968.

16. Ing, M. R.: Early surgical alignment for congenital esotropia. Trans. Am. Ophthalmol. Soc. 79:625, 1981.

17. Chavasse, F. B.: Worth's Squint, or the Binocular Reflexes and the Treatment of Strabismus, 7th ed. Philadelphia, Blakiston's, 1939, p. 519.

18. Fisher, N. F., Flom, M. C., and Jampolsky, A.: Early surgery of congenital esotropia. Am. J. Ophthalmol. 65:439, 1968.

19. Worth, C.: Squint. Its Causes, Pathology, and Treatment, 4th ed. Philadelphia, Blakiston's, 1915, p. 54.

Surgical Treatment of Lateral Rectus Muscle Paralysis*

David A. Lee, M.D., John A. Dyer, M.D., Peter C. O'Brien, Ph.D., and J. Zachary Taylor, M.D.

We conducted a retrospective study of 55 cases to investigate the effectiveness of three different surgical procedures (medial rectus muscle recession and lateral rectus muscle resection in 16 cases, the Hummelsheim procedure in 27 cases, and the Jensen procedure in 12 cases) in the treatment of lateral rectus muscle paralysis. All three procedures were equally effective. Shorter duration of lateral rectus muscle paralysis, greater preoperative lateral version, less contracture of the medial rectus muscle, and a traumatic origin for the sixth cranial nerve damage had a significant effect ($P < .05$) on the final results of surgery.

Lateral rectus muscle paralysis is the most common extraocular muscle palsy. The long intracranial course of the sixth cranial nerve and its anatomic vulnerability are often cited as reasons why it is involved in paralytic strabismus more often than the other two oculomotor nerves. The causes of lateral rectus muscle paralysis are varied, the most common being traumatic, neoplastic, vascular, and idiopathic.[1] Methods for surgical correction of the resulting esotropia vary also.

Usually recession of the overacting and unopposed antagonist (medial rectus muscle) is emphasized rather than resection of the paralyzed lateral rectus muscle, because resection of a paralyzed muscle does not restore function. However, muscle transposition procedures may restore some degree of abduction to the paretic eye.

Hummelsheim[2] is credited with originating muscle transposition as the treatment for lateral rectus muscle paralysis. In his procedure, the lateral halves of the superior and inferior recti muscles are disinserted from their origins and attached to the superior and inferior margins of the scleral insertions of the lateral rectus muscle. Jensen[3] modified Hummelsheim's procedure by splitting the superior, lateral, and inferior recti muscles lengthwise, then tying the lateral half of the superior rectus mus-

*Lee, D. A., Dyer, J. A., O'Brien, P. C., and Taylor, J. Z.: Surgical treatment of lateral rectus muscle paralysis. Published with permission from The American Journal of Ophthalmology. 97:511–518, 1984. Copyright by the Ophthalmic Publishing Company.

cle to the superior half of the lateral rectus muscle and tying the lateral half of the inferior rectus muscle to the inferior half of the lateral rectus muscle with nonabsorbable sutures. A small scleral bite 15 mm posterior to the corneoscleral limbus and midway between the two joining muscles may be taken with each suture to prevent the suture from slipping anteriorly. Either of these procedures can be accompanied by recession of the medial rectus muscle. Helveston[4] reviewed the many modifications of these procedures.

We compared the efficacy of the three procedures—recession of the medial rectus muscle and resection of the lateral rectus muscle, the Hummelsheim procedure, and the Jensen procedure—in the treatment of lateral rectus muscle paralysis.

Subjects and Methods

We conducted a retrospective review of the records from all cases in which surgical procedures for treatment of lateral rectus muscle paralysis were performed at the Mayo Clinic by one of us (J.A.D.) between 1957 and 1982. There were 59 such cases; in 55 the procedure had been one of the three under consideration. In the other four cases, the esotropia was treated by complete vertical muscle transpositions, and we excluded these cases from the study.

We measured and analyzed the following variables: age at the time of surgery; sex; cause (traumatic, neoplastic, vascular, idiopathic, or other); eye involved (right, left, or bilateral); duration (from onset of lateral rectus muscle paralysis to surgery, from initial ocular examination here to surgery, from preoperative ocular examination to surgery); length of follow-up (from surgery to first postoperative ocular examination, from surgery to most recent follow-up examination); amount of medial rectus muscle recession; amount of lateral rectus muscle resection; contracture of the medial rectus muscle at the time of surgery (yes, no, or unknown); and status at the time of latest follow-up (alive or dead). We obtained information from four separate ocular examinations (initial examination here, preoperative examination, postoperative examination, and most recent examination) about best corrected visual acuity, lateral version, medial version, results of the cover-uncover test at near and at distance, and deviation (measured in prism diopters) (Table 1).

We analyzed these data statistically for differences associated with each surgical procedure. We used the Wilcoxon rank sum test to compare age, duration, visual acuity, lateral versions, medial versions, amount of medial and lateral rectus muscle recessions and resections, and deviation in prism diopters at near and at distance. The chi-square test was used to compare sex, cause, eye (right or left), results of the cover-uncover test at

Table 1. General Clinical Data

Clinical Data	Recession-Resection Group	Hummelsheim Group	Jensen Group
No. of patients	16	27	12
Mean age (yrs ± 1 S.D.)	44.4 ± 17.5	33.6 ± 18.8	39.8 ± 19.7
Sex			
Male	6	18	8
Female	10	9	4
Cause of paralysis			
Traumatic	4	19	7
Neoplastic	2	4	3
Vascular	2	0	0
Idiopathic	6	4	0
Other	2*	0	2†
Involved eye			
Right	6	16	5
Left	8	7	5
Both	2	4	2
Time from onset of paralysis to surgery (mos)			
Median	22.5	13.0	18.5
Range	8 to 563	4 to 309	4 to 107
Time from surgery to end of follow-up (days)			
Median	230‡	1,824‡	799.5
Range	2 to 3,958	1 to 7,486	23 to 1,976
Status at end of follow-up			
Alive	16	26	11
Dead	0	1	1

*Encephalitis, 1; multiple sclerosis, 1.
†Encephalopathy, 1; post-Hong Kong flu, 1.
‡Difference statistically significant at P = .009.

distance and at near, medial rectus muscle contracture, and status (alive or dead) at the most recent follow-up. We considered a level of $P \leq .05$ to be statistically significant.

Results

Review of the 55 cases disclosed that recession of the medial rectus muscle and resection of the lateral rectus muscle had been done in 16 cases (29%), the Hummelsheim procedure in 27 cases (49%), and the Jensen procedure in 12 cases (22%).

Table 2. Findings at Initial Ocular Examination

Clinical Data	Recession-Resection Group	Hummelsheim Group	Jensen Group
Time from examination to surgery (days)			
Median	79.5*	335.0*	231.5
Range	1 to 498	1 to 4,995	1 to 455
Visual acuity			
Median	20/20	20/20	20/20
Range	20/20 to 20/400	20/20 to 20/400	20/20 to 20/100
Lateral version (0 to −4)			
Median	−3.0†‡	−4.0†	−4.0‡
Range	−4 to −1	−4 to −1	−4 to 0
Medial version (0 to −4)			
Median	0	0	0
Range	0	−1 to 0	−4 to −3
Esotropia by cover-uncover test (prism diopters)			
Median at distance	32.5	40.0	40.0
Range at distance	6 to 90	20 to 115	20 to 120
Median at near	22.5†‡	40.0†	40.0‡
Range at near	0 to 90	16 to 115	20 to 120

*Difference had borderline statistical significance (P = .06).
†Difference was statistically significant (P = .007).
‡Difference was statistically significant (P = .003).

Only the median interval from surgery to latest follow-up showed a statistically significant intergroup difference, being longer in the Hummelsheim group than in the recession-resection group (P = .009). Although the numbers for several other variables appear disparate, statistical analysis showed no significant intergroup difference in age, sex ratio, cause, laterality of involvement, interval from onset of paralysis to surgery, and status at latest follow-up.

Data obtained at the initial and preoperative ocular examinations (Tables 2 and 3) showed no differences between the Hummelsheim and Jensen groups. The recession-resection group had a somewhat longer interval from initial examination to surgery than did the Hummelsheim group (P = .06, borderline significance); and the recession-resection group differed significantly (P < .01) from the Hummelsheim group and the Jensen group in having more lateral version and less esotropia at near during both the initial and preoperative examinations. The three groups had similar visual acuities, similar medial versions, and similar esotropia at distance in the initial and preoperative examinations. None of the

225

Appendix

Table 3. Clinical Findings at Preoperative Ocular Examination

Clinical Data	Recession-Resection Group	Hummelsheim Group	Jensen Group
Time from examination to surgery (days)			
Median	2.5	2.0	1.5
Range	1 to 80	1 to 84	1 to 42
Visual acuity			
Median	20/20	20/20	20/20
Range	20/20 to 20/400	20/20 to 20/400	20/20 to 20/100
Lateral version (0 to −4)			
Median	−2*†	−4*	−4†
Range	−4 to −1	−4 to −3	−4 to −3
Medial version (0 to −4)			
Median	0	0	0
Range	0	−1 to 0	0
Esotropia by cover-uncover test (prism diopters)			
Median at distance	32.5	50.0	40.0
Range at distance	6 to 50	12 to 115	25 to 120
Median at near	22.5*†	50.0*	40.0†
Range at near	0 to 50	12 to 115	25 to 120

*Difference was statistically significant (P = .002).
†Difference was statistically significant (P = .007).

group values of the measured variables changed significantly from the initial to the preoperative examination in any of the three groups.

Table 4 shows the surgical findings and procedures for the three groups. The median amount of medial rectus muscle recession was 5.25 mm in the recession-resection group, 5.50 mm in the Hummelsheim group, and 7.00 mm in the Jensen group. These differences were significant (P < .01) between the recession-resection and the Jensen groups and between the Hummelsheim and the Jensen groups, but not between the recession-resection and the Hummelsheim groups. The median amount of lateral rectus muscle resection was 7.25 mm for the recession-resection group, 10 mm for the Hummelsheim group, and 0 mm for the Jensen group. These differences were significant (P < .01) for all groups. The amount of medial rectus muscle contracture found at the time of surgery did not differ significantly between any two groups.

None of the 55 patients in this study had anterior segment ischemia resulting from their surgical treatment.

226

Table 4. Surgical Procedures and Observations

Clinical Data	Recession-Resection Group	Hummelsheim Group	Jensen Group
Medial rectus muscle recession (mm)			
Median	5.25*	5.50*	7.00*
Range	2.5 to 10.0	0 to 9.0	6.5 to 10.0
Lateral rectus muscle resection (mm)			
Median	7.25†	10.00†	0†
Range	4.5 to 11.0	2.0 to 13.0	0 to 3.0
Contracture of medial rectus muscle (No. of cases)			
Right			
Yes	3	12	8
No	13	13	4
Unknown	0	0	0
Left			
Yes	7	9	6
No	9	18	6

*Difference was statistically significant ($P < .01$).
†Differences among all groups significant ($P < .01$).

The postoperative and latest recorded ocular examinations (Tables 5 and 6) showed no significant differences between the Hummelsheim and the Jensen groups. At both examinations, lateral version in the recession-resection group was impaired less than in the Hummelsheim group ($P < .001$) and less than in the Jensen group ($P < .001$). Also, at the postoperative examination, medial version in the recession-resection group was significantly less impaired than in the Hummelsheim group ($P = .05$) and less impaired than in the Jensen group ($P = .035$). Otherwise the three groups had similar intervals after surgery, similar visual acuities, and similar results on the cover-uncover test at distance and at near during the postoperative and last examinations. There were no significant group changes from the postoperative to the latest examination.

Because the recession-resection group differed significantly from the Hummelsheim and Jensen groups in lateral version at all four examinations (Tables 2, 3, 5, and 6), it seemed that there might have been a tendency to select patients with less impairment of lateral version for treatment by recession and resection. Attempting to eliminate this selection bias, we excluded those patients in all three groups with preoperative version better than -4. After this correction had been made (No. = 36),

Appendix

Table 5. Clinical Findings at Postoperative Examination

Clinical Data	Recession-Resection Group	Hummelsheim Group	Jensen Group
Time from surgery to examination (days)			
Median	43.5	34.0	33.0
Range	1 to 299	1 to 286	2 to 337
Visual acuity			
Median	20/20	20/20	20/20
Range	20/20 to 20/400	20/20 to 20/400	20/20 to 20/100
Lateral version (0 to −4)			
Median	−1*	−3*	−3*
Range	−4 to 0	−4 to −1	−4 to −1
Medial version (0 to −4)			
Median	−0.5†‡	−1†	−1‡
Range	−1 to 0	−2 to 0	−3 to 0
Cover-uncover test (No. of cases)			
Distance			
Orthophoria	8	16	5
Esotropia	5	6	3
Exotropia	0	3	0
Esophoria	2	0	2
Exophoria	1	2	1
Hyperphoria	0	0	1
Near			
Orthophoria	7	13	7
Esotropia	4	5	1
Exotropia	0	3	2
Esophoria	2	0	2
Exophoria	2	5	0
Hyperphoria	1	1	0

*Difference was statistically significant (P < .001).
†Difference was of borderline significance (P = .05).
‡Difference was statistically significant (P = .035).

analysis of data from the postoperative and the most recent examinations showed no significant difference between any of the surgical groups.

Comparison of data from the preoperative examination and the most recent examination, with and without the correction for selection bias, showed that both lateral version and the results of the cover-

228

Table 6. Clinical Findings at Most Recent Examination

Clinical Data	Recession-Resection Group	Hummelsheim Group	Jensen Group
Time from surgery to examination (mos)			
Median	6.95	11.00	15.68
Range	0.07 to 131.93	0.03 to 221.73	0.77 to 61.63
Visual acuity			
Median	20/20	20/20	20/25
Range	20/20 to 20/400	20/20 to 20/400	20/15 to 20/100
Lateral version (0 to −4)			
Median	−1*	−3*	−4*
Range	−4 to 0	−4 to 0	−4 to −2
Medial version (0 to −4)			
Median	0	−1	−1
Range	−2 to 0	−2 to 0	−4 to 0
Cover-uncover test (No. of cases)			
Distance			
Orthophoria	10	16	6
Esotropia	6	8	3
Esophoria	0	1	3
Exophoria	0	2	0
Near			
Orthophoria	9	13	9
Esotropia	5	7	3
Exotropia	0	2	0
Exophoria	1	5	0
Hyperphoria	1	0	0

*Difference was statistically significant $(P = .001)$.

uncover test at near and at distance improved in all three groups, but medial version worsened mildly in all three groups.

Significant correlations were found between several variables. Preoperative lateral version was correlated negatively with contracture of the medial rectus muscle, which in turn was associated positively with duration of lateral rectus muscle paralysis. Postoperative lateral version was associated positively with preoperative lateral version and was associated negatively with contracture of the medial rectus muscle and duration of lateral rectus muscle paralysis. The surgery effected improvement of lateral version more frequently in cases caused by trauma than in those caused by neoplasm (Table 7).

Table 7. Preoperative Factors Associated (P < .05) with
Postoperative Improvement in Lateral Version

Preoperative Factor	No. of Cases	Lateral Version Improved	
		No.	%
Lateral version −3 or better	19	19	100
Lateral version −4	36	21	58
Cause of paralysis*			
Trauma	26	18	69
Tumor	7	1	14
Duration of paralysis			
Less than 2 yrs	28	18	64
2 yrs or more	8	3	38
Contracture of medial rectus muscle			
No	8	7	88
Yes	28	14	50

*In three cases neither trauma nor tumor caused the paralysis.

Discussion

Several surgical procedures have been proposed for the correction of the esotropia and the lateral rectus muscle weakness or paralysis resulting from damage to the sixth cranial nerve. Our retrospective study suggested that maximal medial rectus muscle recession and lateral rectus muscle resection, the Hummelsheim procedure, and the Jensen procedure may be equally effective in the surgical treatment of lateral rectus muscle paralysis. We found no significant differences in the results of these three procedures.

Several preoperative factors were associated with the outcome of the different procedures. Apparently a longer duration of lateral rectus muscle paralysis allows greater contracture of the medial rectus muscle, resulting in greater preoperative and postoperative impairment of lateral version. This problem might be avoided by performing the surgical correction within two years after the onset of the paralysis. The likelihood of recovering lateral version is less if the sixth-nerve paralysis is caused by a tumor. This is probably because of the destructive nature of the lesion or the greater damage sustained in treatment (surgery or radiation) of the neoplasm.

Although there are clearly limitations inherent in any retrospective study, this report and our clinical experience supported our conclusion that the best surgical treatment for lateral rectus muscle paralysis is a maximal (7 mm) recession of the medial rectus muscle. A moderate (6 to 8 mm) resection of the lateral rectus muscle may be added for a stabilizing effect. The recession-resection procedure is preferable to the more complicated Hummelsheim and Jensen procedures.

References

1. Rush, J. A., and Younge, B. R.: Paralysis of cranial nerves III, IV, and VI. Cause and prognosis in 1,000 cases. Arch. Ophthalmol. 99:76, 1981.
2. Hummelsheim, E.: Weitere Erfahrungen mit partieller Sehnenüberpflanzung an den Augenmuskeln. Arch. Augenheilkd. 62:71, 1909.
3. Jensen, C. D. F.: Rectus muscle union. A new operation for paralysis of the rectus muscles. Trans. Pac. Coast Otoophthalmol. Soc. 45:359, 1964.
4. Helveston, E. M.: Muscle transposition procedures. Surv. Ophthalmol. 16:92, 1971.

Ocular Muscle Surgery in Graves' Disease[*]

John A. Dyer, M.D.

Graves[1] and Von Basedow[2] are credited with the first publications describing the association between thyroid disease and exophthalmos (1835 and 1840). As Wybar[3] has stated, there is still no true understanding of the basic nature of the exophthalmic process. More advanced tests and accurate clinical techniques have been developed to confirm the diagnosis of Graves' disease, but the underlying causative factors thought by many to be autoimmune in nature or abnormalities in cell-mediated immunity have yet to be confirmed or corrected.[4] The thrust of the treatment regimen still is directed toward amelioration of symptoms and, in many cases, subsequent surgical correction of the disabling exophthalmos, ocular muscle imbalance, or eyelid malfunctions which eventuate.

Purpose

The purpose of this paper is to compare the surgical experience in 116 patients who had ocular muscle surgery for Graves' ophthalmopathy between 1968 and 1975[5] with that in 83 new patients operated on subsequently from 1975 through 1977. Some additional surgical procedures that have proved effective will be discussed.

Pathophysiology

In 1969, Werner[6] published a classification of the eye changes of Graves' disease which has been widely accepted:

0 No signs or symptoms
1 Only signs, no symptoms (signs = upper eyelid retraction and stare, with or without lid lag and proptosis)

*Dyer, J. A.: Ocular muscle surgery in Graves' disease. Trans. Am. Ophthalmol. Soc. 76:125–139, 1978. (By permission.)

2 Soft tissue involvement (symptoms and signs = eyelid edema, chemosis, congestion)
3 Proptosis
4 Extraocular muscle involvement
5 Corneal involvement
6 Sight loss (optic nerve involvement)

In this discussion, classes 4 and 6 are of prime interest.

Although many authors believed that the hypotropia and reduced abduction of the eyes were the result of a "paralysis" of the superior rectus and possibly the inferior oblique muscles,[7-10] other reports[5,11-13] confirm that there is, in fact, a fibrosis of the inferior and medial muscles which prevents elevation and abduction through a "leash" effect. This finding led Braley[11] to report a change in intraocular pressure on up-gaze in a number of patients. This, too, has been confirmed.[5] A false diagnosis of glaucoma can be avoided by measuring the intraocular pressure with the eyes in down-gaze or in a relaxed position.

Studies of orbital tissues and ocular muscles in Graves' ophthalmopathy[14,15] indicate that the muscles are enlarged and rubbery and that the orbital fat is under increased tension. Histologically, these changes result from interstitial edema caused by an increase in mucopolysaccharides and round cell infiltration (lymphocytes, plasma cells, macrophages, and mast cells). The presence of these inflammatory cells suggests an immunologic basis for this reaction.

Diagnostic Aids

Electromyographic studies[16-18] have been inconclusive as to whether the basic ocular muscle defect is myogenic or neurogenic. On the other hand, both A-scan and B-scan ultrasonography[5,19-22] have demonstrated the presence of thickened extraocular muscles and, in conjunction with the sophisticated but more costly computerized tomography (CT scan),[5,23,24] have shown clear-cut evidence of enlarged muscles and proptosis. Saccadic velocity studies[25] give further affirmative evidence of a mechanical, restrictive basis for limitation of ocular movement; there is a normal tracing but a terminal slowing of the eye movement (rubber-band effect),[26] whereas in other restrictive situations (blow-out fracture with muscle entrapment, for example) there is a sudden leash effect. Clinically, the forced-duction test and restricted rotations are final confirmation of the restrictive nature of ocular muscle involvement.

Surgical Considerations

The taut fibrous ocular muscles found during a surgical procedure in patients with Graves' myopathy present a unique test of the surgeon's patience and skill. Because of the inflammatory nature of the disease, postoperative scarring often is excessive and a result that looks promising hours or days postoperatively may change to an overcorrection, a regression to the previous state, or the appearance of an entirely new muscle imbalance as weeks pass. Hence, the patient must be apprised of the fact that a second or third or even more procedures may be required. The primary goal is to achieve some degree of single binocular vision in the primary and reading positions; full rotations rarely are achieved.

Basically, the operation of choice is to relax the fibrous, restrictive ocular muscles—most frequently the inferior rectus muscles, secondly the medial recti, less often the superior muscles, and seldom the lateral recti. Some surgeons suggest complete severance of the scleral insertion (inferior muscles), whereas others recess 6 mm or more[27] as a standard procedure; others suggest a graded recession depending on the severity of restriction[5] or an adjustable suture technique,[28-30] so that a muscle can be advanced or recessed several hours postoperatively. This variety of opinions attests to the fact that there is still no panacea for surgical cure of the muscle imbalance. In my experience, reoperation is required in about 40% of patients (Table 1).

Unless very careful and thorough dissection is done along the inferior rectus as far posteriorly as possible to relax or strip away the aponeurosis from the inferior rectus to the lower border of the tarsus, retraction of the lower eyelid may require later surgery (scleral graft). In my experience, any recession more than 4 or 5 mm will result in this complication unless dissection is meticulous. A sharpened lid expressor (Weck) is an ideal instrument for separating these tissues meticulously in any muscle procedure. A large recession (that is, more than 5 mm) was my choice formerly;[5] however, although a complete myectomy or a large recession will relieve the hypotropia or esotropia, it also will create an inability to depress the eyes into the reading position (inferior recti) or will reduce convergence (medial recti) so that bifocals are rendered useless or the patient must hold objects upward in front of his eyes to read. This is particularly annoying when an operation is done on only one inferior muscle.

Other complications, such as exposure of the globes, may occur after the release of fibrotic ocular muscles with an increase in proptosis. In my opinion, if the proptosis is more than 22 or 23 mm (Hertel or Krahn exophthalmometer) serious consideration must be given to orbital decompression before muscle surgery even if there is no threat to vision. The patient should be advised that about 50% of those with no ocular

Table 1.   Ocular Muscle Surgery in Graves' Disease: Patient Profile and Analysis of Surgical Data

	Group 1 (1968–1975)	Group 2 (1975–1977)
No. of patients	116	83
Sex		
Female	85 (73%)	60 (72%)
Male	31 (27%)	23 (28%)
Age (yr)		
Female patients		
Youngest	23	16
Oldest	74	73
Average	51	46
Male patients		
Youngest	26	24
Oldest	75	71
Average	48	49
Orbital decompression		
Total	68 (59%)	57 (69%)
Bilateral		
Transantral	63 (93%)	57 (100%)
Transfrontal	3	0
Combined	2	0
Secondary to muscle surgery	2	1
No. of operations		
1	64 (55%)	52 (63%)
2	33 (29%)	20 (24%)
≥ 3	19 (16%)	11 (13%)
Scleral grafts		
Primary	0	3 (4%)
Secondary	17 (15%)	7 (8%)
Muscles operated primarily		
Inferior and medial only	35 (30%)	46 (55%)
Inferior recti only	48 (41%)	1 (1%)
Other combinations	33 (28%)	36 (43%)
1 inferior only		12 (14%)
Both medial, 1 inferior		8 (10%)
Both inferior, 1 medial		7 (8%)
Medial and inferior, 1 eye		6 (7%)
One medial only		2
Medial muscle only		1

muscle imbalance before decompression will have diplopia afterward and that if an imbalance is present before decompression, it will remain or be more severe after surgery.

The prime indications for orbital decompressions are diplopia with proptosis more than 22 to 23 mm, exposure of the globe, cosmesis, and progressive visual loss because of optic neuropathy. In any patient, a surgical procedure is not advised until the thyroid state is stable. Our otolaryngologists perform the transantral decompressions and anticipate from 2 to 10 mm regression in proptosis. A bilateral procedure always is done to prevent asymmetry. Muscle surgery is delayed four months or longer to permit any ocular muscle change to occur and all tissue reaction to subside.

If only one inferior or medial rectus muscle is involved with minimal proptosis, a recession of the single muscle may suffice. After decompression, most patients require an operation on both inferior and medial muscles; this should be done as one procedure. From experience, I have found that a minimum recession usually suffices because the eye or eyes will elevate or abduct more as times passes. To relax muscles further secondarily is much simpler than to repair an overcorrection. My results are best when recession of the medial rectus muscle is a standard 5 mm and recession of the inferior muscles is varied from 2 to 5 mm so that the pupillary light reflexes from the operating room light are slightly above center in each eye while the patient is under anesthesia. This smaller recession permits the eyes to elevate adequately, yet depression is maintained for satisfactory reading. Jampolsky,[28] Flynn,[29] and Knapp[30] have advocated the use of an adjustable suture—that is, once the muscle is released, the suture arms are passed through the original insertion close together (no scleral bite) and fastened with a slipknot or bow so that some hours later the suture may be tightened or relaxed to improve the eye position. Usually a maximum recession is performed and the muscle is advanced if necessary. Because the postoperative course is so variable in Graves' disease, I have found the variable recession technique best thus far. I do agree that attaching the suture at the original insertion only permits a more normal alignment of the muscle. Vicryl or Dexon sutures of 5-0 or 6-0 caliber are preferred; the tensile strength is excellent, and the tissue reaction is minimal.

Many patients have a definite "A" pattern esotropia. Elevation and abduction of the eyes may be poor; the chin is tilted upward so that single vision can be obtained, and on up-gaze the eyes converge excessively. In the past, I attributed this to the taut inferior muscles failing to relax;[5] however, during surgery I noted that, in many patients, the upper half of the medial muscles often was very thick and swollen whereas the inferior portion was very fibrous and tight, as are the inferior muscles. Subsequently, in these patients I have recessed the lower border of the muscle 2 or 3 mm more than the upper portion and displaced the muscles upward at least one muscle width, as one would do in treating a child with "A" esotropia. Although my experience with these patients has been limited, my impression is that the results are definitely more satisfactory.

From experience I have learned also that a secondary hypertropia is best treated in most instances by a recession of the antagonist superior rectus muscle rather than an advancement of the previously recessed inferior muscle because the problem often is contracture of the superior muscle once the tight inferior muscle is relaxed. If the hyperdeviation is severe, the inferior muscle may require advancement also, but only after weakening of the superior muscle usually a maximum of 4 mm. Because of gradual secondary contracture of the antagonist superior or lateral rectus muscles in this disease, one should postpone further surgical intervention for several months. If the inferior muscle is permitted at surgery to retract freely with no measured recession, its secondary recovery is virtually impossible.

In severe cases in which a large recession is desired primarily or in subsequent operations if further relaxation is desired, proper alignment of the muscles often is difficult. The use of homologous sclera as an extension to the muscle has proved useful.[5] The graft is cut the desired length and width, attached to the distal end of the muscle, covered by a Supramid sleeve, and attached to the original insertion. This ensures a proper alignment of tissue, blends well with muscle and sclera, and permits easy recovery at a later date if needed. The use of Supramid sleeves and caps, as advocated by Knapp[31] and others,[32] is a useful adjunct in secondary procedures especially.

If lower or upper eyelid retraction results in undue exposure of the eyes, surgery designed to correct these defects is in order. This always follows extraocular muscle surgery inasmuch as excessive upper eyelid retraction may result from the patient's thwarted effort to look up and is reduced when the fibrotic inferior muscles are relaxed.

At the Mayo Clinic, a team approach has proved most satisfactory. This team includes an endocrinologist who certifies that the patient's disease is quiescent, an ophthalmologist, and an otolaryngologist who performs the transantral decompressions on the advice of the ophthalmologist; at least two of these team members must examine the patient and suggest decompression for reasons previously discussed. Afterward, ocular muscle surgery and subsequent eyelid realignment are performed if needed.

Clinical Experience

In a previous paper,[5] I reported my experience with ocular muscle surgery in 116 patients operated on from 1968 to 1975. The following is a comparison of these results with the results in 83 patients who had surgery from 1975 through 1977 (Table 1). All of these patients were operated on by me, and none of the last group had had surgery in prior years.

In both groups, the female population was about three-fourths the total number. The average age of female patients was 51 years in group 1 and 46 years in group 2. The average age of male patients was 48 years in group 1 and 49 years in group 2. Orbital decompression was performed before muscle surgery in 68 patients (59%) of group 1, 63 (93%) of these having a transantral decompression. In comparison, 57 patients (69%) of group 2 had a decompression and all had a transantral procedure. Decompression was done secondary to muscle surgery in two patients in group 1 and in one patient in group 2. Sixty-four (55%) of those in group 1 had a single surgical procedure compared with 52 (63%) of those in group 2, whereas two procedures were done in 33 patients (29%) in group 1 and in 20 patients (24%) in group 2. Three or more procedures were done in 16% of group 1 patients and in 13% of group 2 patients. Homologous scleral grafts to extend ocular muscles were used in secondary procedures in 17 patients (15%) of group 1; scleral grafts were used in primary procedures in 3 patients (4%) and in secondary procedures in 7 patients (8%) in group 2. Whereas 35 patients (30%) of group 1 had both inferior and medial muscles operated primarily, 46 patients (55%) of group 2 had this as a first operation. Both inferior muscles were recessed in 48 (41%) of group 1 patients, whereas only 1 patient had this procedure in group 2. Other combinations of muscles were operated in 33 patients (28%) of group 1 and in 36 patients (43%) of group 2.

From this comparison it appears that some progress has been made in decreasing the number of procedures required to achieve single binocular vision for patients with severe muscle imbalance.

Summary

When the thyroid state is stable and no further changes in ocular motility are occurring, surgical correction of diplopia is necessary to regain single vision in the primary and reading positions. Preliminary tests including A-scan and B-scan ultrasonography, the CT scan, saccadic velocity testing, and forced-duction tests aid in excluding other causes of muscle abnormalities.

In the absence of proptosis and with minimal eyelid retraction, recession of the taut rectus muscles, most often the inferior and secondly the medial, is required.

If proptosis is moderate (22 to 23 mm) and lid retraction is severe, preliminary orbital decompression (bilateral transantral) is advised inasmuch as prior relaxation of the ocular muscles may cause increased proptosis and exposure of the eyes, which would necessitate emergency orbital decompression.

If severe proptosis creates a cosmetic blemish, or if exposure of the globes or optic neuropathy is a threat to vision, decompression should be done, followed in four months or longer by ocular muscle surgery. After decompression, diplopia may occur in almost 50% of patients with no muscle imbalance preoperatively , whereas all patients with diplopia before decompression will have a more severe imbalance after decompression.

Although I advocated larger recessions of the fibrotic muscles previously,[5] a smaller, graded recession of the inferior muscles after careful dissection is more accurate and prevents lower eyelid retraction. Transposition of the medial muscles upward with recession is helpful in many patients with an "A" pattern esotropia. With time, the antagonist superior rectus muscle contracts and must be recessed secondarily if a large inferior recession has resulted in overcorrection. Advancement of the inferior muscle(s) will not suffice. The use of scleral grafts to extend the ocular muscles and placement of Supramid sleeves or caps are useful adjuncts in reoperations.

These findings have led to a decrease in the number of surgical procedures required to gain useful single vision for these patients. As a general rule, if the pupillary light reflexes from the operating room light are almost centered in each eye at the conclusion of surgery, the eyes will remain in this position when the patient awakens. Because of the fibrotic state of the muscles, full rotations seldom are regained.

When the thyroid state is stable, relieve the proptosis, straighten the eyes, and correct the eyelid retraction for most effective results.

References

1. Graves RJ: Clinical lectures. *London Med Surg J* 7:516, 1835.
2. Von Basedow KA: Exophthalmus durch hypertrophie des Zellgewebes in der Augenhöhle, *Wchnschr Heilk Berl* 6:197; 220, 1840.
3. Wybar KC: The nature of endocrine exophthalmos. *Bibl Ophthalmol* 49:119, 1957.
4. Gorman CA: The presentation and management of endocrine ophthalmopathy. *Clin Endocrinol Metabol* 7:67, 1978.
5. Dyer JA: The oculorotary muscles in Graves' disease. *Trans Am Ophthalmol Soc* 74:425, 1976.
6. Werner SC: Classification of thyroid disease: report of the committee on nomenclature (letter to editor). *J Clin Endocrinol Metab* 29:860, 1969.
7. Rundle FF, Wilson CW: Ophthalmoplegia in Graves' disease. *Clin Sci* 5:17, 1944.
8. Brain R: The diagnosis, prognosis and treatment of endocrine exophthalmos. *Trans Ophthalmol Soc UK* 82:223, 1962.

9. Grob D: Myopathies and their relation to thyroid disease. *NY State J Med* 63:218, 1963.

10. Goldstein JE: Paresis of superior rectus muscle: associated with thyroid dysfunction. *Arch Ophthalmol* 72:5, 1964.

11. Braley AE: Malignant exophthalmos. *Am J Ophthalmol* 36:1286, 1953.

12. Miller JE: Acquired strabismus in adults. *South Med J* 54:744, 1961.

13. Miller JE, van Heuven W, Ward R: Surgical correction of hypotropias associated with thyroid dysfunction. *Arch Ophthalmol* 74:509, 1965.

14. Kroll AJ, Kuwabara T: Dysthyroid ocular myopathy: anatomy, histology, and electron microscopy. *Arch Ophthalmol* 76:244, 1966.

15. Riley FC: Orbital pathology in Graves' disease. *Mayo Clin Proc* 47:975, 1972.

16. Magora A, Chaco J, Zauberman H: An electromyographic investigation of ophthalmoplegia in thyrotoxicosis. *Arch Ophthalmol* 79:170, 1968.

17. Schultz RO, Van Allen MW, Blodi FC: Endocrine ophthalmoplegia: with an electromyographic study of paretic extraocular muscles. *Arch Ophthalmol* 63:217, 1960.

18. Breinen GM: New aspects of ophthalmoneurologic diagnosis. *Arch Ophthalmol* 58:375, 1957.

19. Coleman DJ, Jack RL, Franzen LA, Werner SC: High resolution B-scan ultrasonography of the orbit. V. Eye changes of Graves' disease. *Arch Ophthalmol* 88:465, 1972.

20. Werner SC, Coleman DJ, Franzen LA: Ultrasonographic evidence of a consistent orbital involvement in Graves' disease. *N Engl J Med* 290:1447, 1974.

21. Ossoinig K: Echo-orbitography: a reliable method for the differential diagnosis of endocrine exophthalmos. In *Further Advances in Thyroid Research*. Vol 2. Edited by K Fellinger, R Höfer: Wien, G. Gistel & Cie, 1971, p 871.

22. Forrester JV, Sutherland GR, McDougall IR: Dysthyroid ophthalmopathy: orbital evaluation with B-scan ultrasonography. *J Clin Endocrinol Metab* 45:221, 1977.

23. Kriss JP, Marshall WH Jr, Enzmann DR, Rosenthal AR: Computed axial tomography of the orbit in patients with Graves' ophthalmopathy. *Excerpta Medica International Congress Series* 378:621, 1975.

24. Hodes BL, Weinberg P: A combined approach for the diagnosis of orbital disease: computed tomography and standardized A-scan echography. *Arch Ophthalmol* 95:781, 1977.

25. Metz HS: Saccadic velocity studies in patients with endocrine ocular disease. *Am J Ophthalmol* 84:695, 1977.

26. Mims J: Saccadic velocity analysis (lecture). Florida Midwinter Seminar, Boca Raton, Florida, February 5–8, 1978.

27. Schimek RA: Surgical management of ocular complications of Graves' disease. *Arch Ophthalmol* 87:655, 1972.

28. Jampolsky A: Personal communication.

29. Flynn J: Personal communication.

30. Knapp P: Personal communication.

31. Knapp P: Personal communication.

32. Dunlap EA: Plastic implants in muscle surgery: plastic materials in the management of extraocular motility restrictions. *Arch Ophthalmol* 80:249, 1968.

Discussion

DR PHILIP KNAPP. I want to thank Doctor Dyer for handing me this paper almost two months ago in Honolulu. It is fortunate for me that he did as I just got back from the Far East the night before last.

As you just heard, the author has described what is known about the orbital changes in Graves' disease and he has listed all the fancy and expensive tests available to make the diagnosis. However, as far as the disturbances in ocular motility are concerned, these tests are rarely needed, for the diagnosis is clinical. Nothing else looks like it or acts like it. Moreover, the traction test cinches the diagnosis.

I think the number of cases presented by Doctor Dyer is most impressive. The increase from 113 cases in over 7 years to 83 in the next three years leads to one of two conclusions. Either the Mayo Clinic has built a better mouse trap or the team has gotten more confident so that they are operating on a higher percentage of patients. Certainly, the figure that 69% have had a bilateral orbital decompression by the Ogura method is startling. Our figure is only 10% but we reserve this type of decompression for patients needing a sight-saving procedure either due to the danger of exposure of the cornea or to compression of the optic nerves. This 69% producing 50% of new motility disturbances is one of the reasons so many patients require muscle surgery. We have found that 13% of our patients develop new muscle problems following decompression. We think that many of these patients with exophthalmos of only 22–23 mm can be cosmetically relieved by working on the lids—either recessing the levator or by raising the lower lids with a scleral graft. In such patients one should do the lid surgery first because it will not affect the motility, but we entirely agree that muscle surgery should wait until after the orbital decompressions. We feel the Ogura decompression is a formidable procedure with reported complications including blindness. I would like to ask Doctor Dyer whether they have had any significant complications besides the disturbed motility?

The author feels that the inflammatory nature of the process leads to excessive postoperative reaction with the resulting scar tissue causing instability of the operative result. I would agree that the results of muscle surgery in Graves' disease are unstable but feel inflammatory reaction causes only part of them. This part can be minimized by recessing the conjunctiva fully, plus using frequent steroid drops alternating with lubricating drops as exposure contributes to the postoperative reaction. Our orthoptic department and I think that some of the postoperative instability is really a failure to evaluate correctly the preoperative measurements.

As the ocular myopathy involves all the recti muscles though frequently in varying degree, a marked contracture of one vertical rectus may overshadow other involvements, which then become apparent postoperatively. A marked increase or reduction in a hypertropia in a field where one would not expect such a change may indicate involvement of another or other muscles. Operating to correct these discrepancies at the same time as the main culprit may save subsequent operations, particularly if one uses adjustable sutures which I feel are the best method of achieving a variable recession.

I certainly agree with Doctor Dyer that an excessive recession leading to the crippling of the muscle's action is to be avoided. Not only does this lead to a marked limitation of motion in the field of the crippled muscle, but like any paresis it sets up an ideal condition for subsequent contracture of the yoke or direct antagonist.

I have had no experience with the use of homologous sclera to lengthen the muscle further without losing its arc of contact. If one were to do such a procedure, the use of Supramid Extra would certainly be helpful to prevent adhesions from nullifying the effect of surgery. I have merely added a "Z" or marginal myotomy to the recessed muscle to achieve the same lengthening effect without losing the arc of contact.

I have never been aware of the "A" patterns he reports. The patients I have seen showing this have had congenital fibrosis of the inferior rectus rather than Graves' disease. It has been my thought that releasing the taut inferior rectus was all that was necessary, just as recessing the tight lateral rectus stops the upshoot on attempted adduction with a Duane's syndrome.

There is one frustrating aspect in treating these patients that has really upset me. After a successful result with a good field of single binocular vision, a year or two later a deviation occurs. I remember one woman in whom this happened twice. Has the author also had this miserable experience?

Finally, I would like to congratulate the author on this excellent report of his extensive (probably unparalleled) experience in treating this frustrating problem.

Dr John A. Dyer. Thank you, Doctor Knapp. Many of the patients have only a moderate degree of proptosis and minimal exposure problems. When lid retraction is the primary problem and diplopia is not present, we will either do a recession of Mueller's muscle or place a scleral graft in the upper or lower eyelids as a primary and perhaps the only procedure.

As to complications of decompression, we have had only one patient in some 350 who had any problem with vision afterwards. This patient had reduced vision in one eye, probably due to postoperative hemorrhage. The vision returned to normal, as I recall. The remainder of the complications are very minor in nature. One or two patients had a fistula that remained postoperatively; these were closed secondarily.

Some patients have inturning of the lower lids because of a "setting sun" appearance to the eyes after liberal decompressions. The otolaryngologist has become a little less vigorous now. If the entropion is severe, a scleral graft to reduce this may be required at a later date. Other than that, the complications are minimal.

I would agree with Doctor Knapp that clinical testing, especially forced-traction testing, is important. If one excludes trauma, there really is no other muscle involvement quite like Graves' disease. One can diagnose this problem with a forced-traction test. This is especially so at surgery with the patient under anesthesia.

As to ischemic iritis, I have had only one patient who showed some cells and flare and a slight clouding of the cornea in one eye the first postoperative day. The remainder of the patients have not had any problem with ischemic iritis. Some of these muscles are so tight that the pull on the muscle for a sustained period of time results in much pressure on the globe. I think many of these eyes have a hypotony and perhaps some degree of inflammation just from the vigorous manipulation of the globe.

Recurrent problems do occur. The patient may have single binocular vision after surgery for nine months or twelve months and return with a new or added muscle problem, without a flare-up of the Graves' disease. I think this is further evidence that there is some continually progressive inflammatory process in the muscles.

The number of decompressions has increased because a greater number of patients who have more severe Graves' ophthalmopathy have been referred to us. Thank you very much.

Bibliography

Allen, J. H.: Strabismus Ophthalmic Symposium. St. Louis, The C. V. Mosby Company, 1950.

Allen, J. H.: Strabismus Ophthalmic Symposium II. St. Louis, The C. V. Mosby Company, 1958.

Apt, L.: An anatomical reevaluation of rectus muscle insertions. Trans. Am. Ophthalmol. Soc. 78:365–375, 1980.

Bedrossian, E. H.: Surgical and Nonsurgical Management of Strabismus. Springfield, Illinois, Charles C Thomas, 1969.

Breinin, G. M.: The Electrophysiology of Extraocular Muscle: With Special Reference to Electromyography. Toronto, University of Toronto Press, 1962.

Breinin, G. M., Swan, K. C., and Costenbader, F. D.: Symposium: Accommodative esotropia. Trans. Amer. Acad. Ophthal. Otolaryng. 61:375–396 (May-June) 1957.

Dendy, H. M., and Shaterian, E. T.: Practical Ocular Motility. Springfield, Illinois, Charles C Thomas, 1967.

Duke-Elder, W. S.: Clinical Surgery: The Eye. Vol. 2. London, Butterworth & Co., Ltd., 1964.

Fink, W. H.: Surgery of the Vertical Muscles of the Eye. Ed. 2. Springfield, Illinois, Charles C Thomas, 1962.

Gibson, G. G., and Harley, R. D.: Anomalies of Binocular Position, Visual Perception and Ocular Motility in Strabismus. Rochester, Minnesota, American Academy of Ophthalmology and Otolaryngology, 1966.

Helveston, E. M.: Atlas of Strabismus Surgery. Ed. 2. St. Louis, C. V. Mosby Company, 1977.

Lyle, T. K., and Bridgeman, G. J. O.: Worth and Chavasse's Squint: The Binocular Reflexes and the Treatment of Strabismus. Ed. 9. London, Baillière, Tindall & Cox, 1959.

Ogle, K. N., Martens, T. G., and Dyer, J. A.: Oculomotor Imbalance in Binocular Vision and Fixation Disparity. Philadelphia, Lea & Febiger, 1967.

Parks, M. M., and Parker, J. E.: Atlas of Strabismus Surgery. Philadelphia, Harper & Row, Publishers, 1983.

Schlossman, A., and Priestley, B. S.: Strabismus. Int. Ophthal. Clin. 6:1–749 (Fall) 1966.

Sugar, H. S.: The Extrinsic Eye Muscles. Rochester, Minnesota, American Academy of Ophthalmology and Otolaryngology, 1947.

Von Noorden, G. K., and Maumenee, A. E.: Atlas of Strabismus. St. Louis, The C. V. Mosby Company, 1967.

Index

Note: Page numbers in *italics* refer to
illustrations. Page numbers in **boldface**
refer to tables.

Index